# Diet Sm

# 10-DAY GR                    E

# CLEANSE:

*Lose up to10 pounds and10 years in just 10 days*
*Could this be your last diet and weight loss book?*

## Marcus D. Norman
## Dr. George Della Pietra

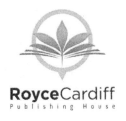

**Royce**Cardiff
Publishing House

Copyright © 2014

First-Edition

ISBN-13: 978-0692461372 (Royce Cardiff Publishing House)

ISBN-10: 069246137X

Printed in the United States of America

MarcusDNorman@gmail.com

## DEDICATION

*To my father, you inspired me in more ways than you will ever know*

# CONTENTS

## Why This Detox and Weight Loss Program?

Welcome! I'm excited for you. You have just taken your first step to being free of weight gain and poor health issues.

You deserve to and are designed to live your life as healthy and happy as possible. The reason I and Dr. George Della Pietra put this book together was to help as many people as possible. To let you realize it's not your fault, and show you how you can turn away from this epidemic of excess weight and poor health issues.

The five basic steps in this book will take you a long way beyond just losing a few pounds.

- We're going to show you how to keep it off. No more yo-yo diets and fluctuating weights, and no starvation diet either. Been there, done that!

- We're going to introduce you to a diet plan that will satisfy you and give you all that your body needs and more, as well as all-you-can-eat foods! Really, it's very delicious!

- Lifestyle changes that you can follow easily, that will promote you to feeling great, thinking clearer, having more stamina and energy, as well as a better sex life! Oh yes!

- The all- round ultimate exercise which is just 10 minutes a day! You need to know about this!

- Why I believe you should not take supplements

- How to look and feel at least ten years younger

This is not just another diet book; this is a step-by-step, easy-to-follow lifestyle changing guide. Do a little or do as much as you like, this book will open up the door for many unaware of the principles inside.

I was 30 pounds overweight and had been diagnosed with incurable diseases, but I had them vanish from my life forever with the five basic steps covered in this book.

If you are reading this book, then you're looking for real answers. Sometimes it can feel hard or even hopeless doing what the experts say. They seem to offer little or no long-lasting results. You experience pain and

i

embarrassment with friends, family, and even strangers, not to mention the loss of money and irreplaceable time. I know this because I have been there.

If the suggested steps in this book help you, please pass this information on to other people who could benefit from it.

I would love to hear from you!

If you would like to contact Dr. George Della Pietra or Myself Marcus D Norman with any success stories, or would like to be put on our free life changing health book list when they are available. Please contact us at MarcusDNorman@gmail.com

Wishing you an even happier and healthy life!

ii

# Chapter 1

## Do You Think It Is Possible to Lose 10 Pounds and 10 Years in 10 Days?

- Can I really lose the stubborn pounds and keep them off?
- Can I look and feel fabulous, be sexier, be energized and not get sick anymore?
- Can I make a permanent weight loss and health improvement?

The short answer is YES!

Please allow me to explain. There are historical and scientific data that have been proven over and over again by hundreds of thousands of people. Some of these data even go as far back as 250,000 years ago!

In the following chapters were going to explain.

- Why it's not your fault
- Why it's not about you or your body
- How to stop the fad starvation yo-yo diets and eat all that you want.

Did you know Dr. George Della Pietra has reduced or eliminated incurable diseases with a similar program covered in this book?

There are two medical and scientific facts you must know, and once you know and understand these facts and know how to correct them, your whole well-being will change in a short time, forever.

By making changes and corrections, not only will you find your ideal weight, the bonus is you very well may reduce or eliminate discomfort, sicknesses and diseases in your life. I once told Dr. George how amazing that was, his reply was its just knowledge and science, and it's not magic.

Almost anybody can follow this step-by-step guide, all the information you need never to have to go through another diet or weight loss plan ever again is included. There are gentle baby steps, modifications and suggestions for those that want it. Enclosed are over 100 quick and easy to make superfood green smoothie recipes.

You can start receiving healthy energizing benefits starting today (see chapter 4).

Is it possible to lose 10 pounds and 10 years in 10 days? The answer is incontrovertible YES! as it has been accomplished by hundreds of thousands of people before you. When your health is where it should be, you will feel more fantastic, full of life, have stamina and be a better lover.

You don't think your weight problems are your fault? You're right, we will go over scientific facts that you need to know, and what you can do about it. In this book, Dr. George Della Pietra offers his medical expertise on how he cures his patients and how to permanently turn around your whole health. Can you do this? This is a step-by-step guide, most people do just fine, and, however, for those who require adjustments or modifications, they are suggested in the book.

*"The doctor of the future will no longer treat the human frame with drugs, but rather will cure and prevent disease with nutrition."*

-Thomas Edison

## Chapter 2

## Do You Know That Being Overweight and Unhealthy Is Not Your Fault in Its Entirety?

It has nothing to do with your genes or your family history, don't buy into the modern concept; it's just a scapegoat to blame somebody else or an excuse to give you another pill. It's all about your diet, please allow me to explain.

We are going to cover three major causes of weight gain, health issues and feeling poor; we're also going to talk about the steps you can take to reverse it.

The first thing we're going to discuss is something that is present in nearly 80% of the food you eat today if you eat like the average person. Its corn, and corn is a killer. Don't throw arrows and knives at me at this moment, please let me explain. 30 years ago, if you were like me and you lived on or near a farm, you most likely ate wonderful, fresh table corn, delicious, beautiful, healthy stuff. The corn I am referring to is our modern day food stock corn. For one example, 30 to 40 years ago, a good yield was 40 bushels per acre of good, table eating corn. However, in recent times, farms can yield up to 180 to 200 bushels per acre of feedstock corn that is not for your dining table. That is phenomenal.

The benefit to humankind is that it creates cheap food. As a matter of fact, that was the intention, it is something being purposefully carried out by the American government and the farmers. America and many First World countries now spend a lot less of their hard earned money on food than our grandparents did just a few decades back. For example, an average American spends about 16% to 18% of his/her money on food, while our grandparents spent 25 to 50%. Factually, many Third World countries still spend a lot more on food. So we are rich, we live like kings and queens. Our forefathers who founded our countries spent most of their days finding, harvesting, hunting, just to feed their families. Today we are blessed, overabundant is the norm and we can buy several varieties of foods from all around the world at a very reasonable price.

**The Hidden Cost of Cheap Food:**

There is one thing that is present in 80% of your food, which you should not consume.

The corn industry, approximately 40 years ago had a glut of corn. Millions were spent to research and find out other markets for the product. They came up with corn syrup, sounds harmless enough doesn't it. Within 12 years, the majority of the sweeteners in all of our foods and drinks had been replaced with corn syrup. The issue is that this type of corn is void of nutrients, and there are studies that prove that it is not only void of nutrients, it is harmful to us.

This type of corn is called feedstock corn, and it is mostly what goes into feeding livestock such as chickens, pigs, and cows. Cows can, for example, be fed grain (which primarily consists of corn) for the last 140 days of their lives in order to effectively fatten them up for better profit. You ever heard of the term grain fed? We all used to believe that was a good thing. However, it is important that you realize that this type of diet is not natural

3

for the cows, as they can get very sick and have digestive issues or ulcers. As consumers, it is not an ideal protein source.

The other primary use for this type of corn feedstock is to make corn syrup. It makes for very cheap sugar, and manufacturers choose it because it's very cost-effective. Test it out for yourself next time you're in the grocery store. Walk up any aisle and see for yourself how many products contain corn syrup or some corn type of product, you may be shocked. Remember, this type of corn possesses no nutritional value, has empty calories, hence, and is detrimental to your health.

**People who drink one can of soda per day double their chances of being a diabetic.**

Solution:

The obvious solution is to stop eating foods with this void nutritional sugar. In later chapters, we will give you an excellent, delicious, wholesome energizing foods to replace them with. Have no worries.

TEN-DAY GREEN SUPERFOOD SMOOTHIE CLEANSE

### Factory Food, Plastic Food!

Food manufacturers a long time ago discovered how to make profitable foods. The only problem, however, was that many of the foods had very little or no flavor at all! They eventually found a solution. If they put these four ingredients in the food, your body will always give you the signal that it's not satisfied yet, so you still feel hungry, and you are compelled to eat more. You should know that your body never gives you the signal to stop because your nutritional needs have not yet been met. The four ingredients are:

- Fat
- Sugar
- Salt
- MSG

The formula for making a lot of money in the food industry is- cheap cost to make. It's not necessary to have flavor because if you add in enough fat, sugar, salt and MSG, it will have your customers coming back for more.

Good for business, but not your body!

Since these products lack nutritional value and are devoid of any of life, they ultimately have a long shelf life that is even better for business. The simple solution is to make other choices that serve your health.

Can you see how overeating is not your fault? If you're eating foods that you think tastes great, and your body signals are telling you it is not nutritionally full yet. Which keeps you hungry, and wanting more, so you continue to eat. You logically are not in control of the quantities you are consuming. Have you ever noticed when you ate something really healthy like a salad, carrot juice or fresh fruits and veggies, and you realized you just didn't feel hungry? This is because you were nutritionally satisfied. To reinforce my point, can you continually eat and eat and eat and eat salad at one serving? No right? It's very difficult. However, with potato chips, I could devour a whole, large one-pound bag by myself, nearly biting off the hand of anybody who would stick their fingers in my bag, if you know what I mean.

I used to binge in front of the TV and eat one-pound bags of chocolate M&Ms and a can of Coca-Cola. The funny thing is I knew I would feel terrible later, but I would continually eat until the bag was empty. Sometimes, I would even go so far as to turn the movie off, drive to the store and buy another bag! Do you think food can be addictive? Believe me, it's not your fault.

**Two Simple Truths:**

In a nutshell, here's the simple reason our world today is in such a medical mess, why people are getting sicker and older.

Statistics has revealed that this next young generation may live shorter lives than their parents.

This is the first of such in recorded history.

- Toxic buildup = toxic chemicals in food, drugs
- Unhealthy population = lack of nutrients in our food

Some of our factory foods require more energy from our bodies in order to be processed than we gain. In other words, it's a net loss of energy, and this can leave you hungry, dissatisfied, rundown and vulnerable to sickness. This, in the long run, leads to more drugs (toxins), and can have a long-term downward spiral effect on your health if not stopped. As you can witness about what is going on in the First World Country of today, there are many epidemics of diseases. How many people do you know that have some form of cancer?

**Good News:**

The answer is simple, we need to do the opposite of what we did to get here:

- Flush out the toxins
- Flood your body with easy bio-available nutrients

You will accomplish this with a ten-day superfood green smoothie cleanse. You will feel like you've never felt before, not only that, you will start to notice your mental clarity coming back in the first two or three days.

Here is one of the biggest reasons you should do a superfood smoothie fast. It will reset your body clock. In other words, you will stop craving the junk food that was so cleverly engineered for you to eat; rather, your body will crave healthy foods.

TEN-DAY GREEN SUPERFOOD SMOOTHIE CLEANSE

It's natural to choose healthy foods; my three-year-old daughter has always picked fresh fruits and vegetables over junk food. One of her favorite foods is raw broccoli. How many kids in America would pick broccoli over cookies?

**Stress:**

Stress is a killer, it takes away from the quality of your life, and can keep you from being focused. Not only can it make you no good for yourself, it can also make you no good to your family and friends. Here are some basic stress fixes! (We will cover these in more details later in the book).

**Stress fixes**

- Meditation
- Sleep
- Healthy eating
- Regular good sex, oh yes can we say stress relief!

Could this be the real solution to limiting excess weight and diseases from your life?

It's not your fault, corn syrup, artificial sweeteners, fat, sugar, salt and MSG help you over eat and leave you lacking a proper healthy nutrition. You most likely have a toxic buildup in your system and are not getting enough nutrients in your body. This causes a plethora of health issues, and the results can be weight gain, not feeling well and a general lack of energy. The good news is you can turn this around by avoiding these types of foods and additives, and by doing this ten-day smoothie cleanse (Taking out the trash) which will help flush out the toxins and put bio-available nutrients back in your system, thereby, effectively resetting your body clock. Afterward, you will begin to crave healthy foods. You learned stress is a killer. That the smoothie cleanse, and some of the easy-to-follow steps will equally assist you in reducing stress further on. The bottom line is you have a lot to look forward to now that you have this knowledge. You can see that by limiting a few things and changing a few habits, you can jumpstart a whole new healthy you. No worries, we will cover what to do after this cleanse, and make sure you can continue your incredible journey to a new, happier, and healthier you.

*"Processed food not only extends the shelf life, but they extend the waistline as well."*

--Karen Sessions

Now that you know how to turn your health around and get to your perfect weight let's talk about SAD (Standard American Diet) in the next chapter. How if you do not make any changes in your normal diet, you will most likely die of one of the top 15 diseases way before your time!

# Chapter 3

## Weight Gain and Poor Health Are Symptoms, and Not the Problem.

### Do You Know Your SAD Is Killing You?

SAD = Standard American Diet

If you keep eating the standard American diet, there's a very high chance you will die of one of the top 15 diseases below. You can see for yourself, just look around at your family, friends, and acquaintances, what's happening to them? How many Friends have you lost in the past year to any of these top 15 killers?

> *I wish to remind you that money and wealth are not the most important elements in your life. As you know, without health, the richest man or woman is truly poor. What is today's most serious health hazards are the foods prepared for you by other people. These foods include fast foods, processed supermarket foods, restaurant meals, etc. Most purveyors of commercial foods are only interested in profits, not in providing wholesome foods. Consequentially, expect foods prepared with hydrogenated oils, trans-fats, wrong sugars, artificial sweeteners (the most dangerous one of which is corn syrup — all coal, also called corn sugar), toxic tap water, vegetable sprayed with pesticides and grown with artificial fertilizers, fumigated or genetically modified, feed lot beef, farm raised fish, etc.*
>
> *— Diane Morgan*

### Top 15 Causes of Death in America

Chances are if you follow the historically proven steps outlined in this book, you can prevent about 14 of the top 15 causes of death in the First World. Even though S. A. D. Stands for Standard American Diet,

I like to think of it as **Simply Accepting Death!**

Also included are some incurables diseases and issues that have been helped, reversed or prevented by merely following the outline of this timetested life changing program.

*The top two causes of death are responsible for more than 50 percent of the annual death toll

1. Diseases of the heart
2. Malignant tumors (Cancer)
3. Cerebrovascular diseases
4. Chronic lower respiratory diseases
5. Accidents (unintentional injuries)
6. Diabetes mellitus
7. Influenza and pneumonia
8. Alzheimer's disease
9. Nephritis, nephrotic syndrome, and nephrosis
10. Septicemia (blood poisoning)
11. Suicide
12. Chronic liver disease and cirrhosis
13. Primary hypertension and hypertensive renal disease
14. Parkinson's disease (tied)
15. Homicide (tied)

> *"He who cures a disease may be the skill-fullest,*
> *But he that prevents it is the safest physician."*
> ~ Thomas Fuller

Below is an additional partial, however not exhaustive list of ailments or improvements that have been helped significantly if not entirely reversed.

- Children with ASD, APD, ADHD and SPD
- Herpes
- Candida
- Autoimmune diseases (multiple sclerosis)
- Asthma
- Bodybuilding: Reshaping the body for shaping, toning, and building muscle
  TEN-DAY GREEN SUPERFOOD SMOOTHIE CLEANSE

- Acne

- Anti-aging

- Psoriasis

- Eczema

- HIV/AIDS

- Competitive Sports

- Proper Elimination

- Dental Health and Surgery

- Brain power (increase capacity and clarity)

- Bipolar Syndromes

- Diabetes Type II

- Hair Re-growth

- Recovering from Surgery

- Immune System Builder

- Flu Shot Alternative

- Menstruation Problems

- Paralysis

- Cardiovascular Disease

- Bronchitis

- Constipation

- Arthritis and Joint Pain

- Blood Pressure Issues

- Reproductive Issues

- Skin Pigmentation

- Itching

- Rashes

- Leaky Gut

- Feel-Good Chemistry

As you can see for yourself, there's a long list here, and this is not everything. However, as you can imagine, when you allow the body to be in balance and heal itself, your body will prevent diseases and many possible issues.

I had been diagnosed with two incurable diseases and without the information that I discovered, I surely would not be around today!

## Medical Industry:

I've worked in the medical industry in one of the top 100 facilities in United States, and I can honestly say that there are a lot of wonderful, caring, heartfelt people in this industry. However, the challenge is that most of the information, education, and government laws are manipulated and controlled by the pharmaceutical companies. Unfortunately, I've seen it for myself; a lot of emphasis and focus is placed on profit. There is no profit in it for them if people are dead or healthy, their incentive is for you to not be actually healthy, but just need more of their wonderful little pills. Don't get me wrong, I'm not saying there's no place for modern medicine, it can be amazing if used in the right example. One example is if you had an accident, you may count your blessings and have your life saved by this amazing world of science.

The bottom line is if you continue to eat a SAD diet, you will most likely die of one of the top 15 causes of death. You may have to keep unhappily putting your family and friends out, and spending large amounts of time and money just to have a low-quality existence. I have seen this more than I care to remember. I'm so happy you are reading this. Is this your wake-up call?

## A Solution:

It's obvious you need to stop eating the standard American diet, stop polluting your body. Eat and thrive on nutritionally rich foods, which we will go into in more detail later on in this book.

If you don't change your standard American diet, you will most likely die before your time and not feel superb about it. Pharmaceutical companies have an agenda for profit, and they are the educators of our current medical system. If you change your diet to nutritionally rich foods, your chances of living a long, healthy happy life are greatly increased.

If you would like to get off this addictive degrading lifestyle, get to the next chapter on the fundamental principles, knowledge and understanding of

TEN-DAY GREEN SUPERFOOD SMOOTHIE CLEANSE

what two things to give up so as to maximize your health, happiness, and lifestyle.

> *"The food you eat can be either the safest and most powerful form of medicine or the slowest form of poison."*
>
> ~ Ann Wigmore

*APA: How Stuff Works "15 Most Common Causes of Death in the United ... (n.d.). Retrieved from http://health.howstuffworks.com/diseases-conditions/death-dying/15most-common-causes-of-death-in-the-united-states.htm_br

# Chapter 4

## It Starts with Food
## Five Simple Steps so You Can Create
## Your Perfect Health and Weight

### Are You Ready for a 10 Day Green Superfood Smoothie Challenge?

This is a large chapter, and we have a lot to take in. We will be going over the Following Subjects.

Step 1 Detox

Step 2 Exercise

Step 3 Relaxation Response

Step 4 Whole Superfood and Nutrients

Step 5 Green Superfood Smoothies Fasting

In this chapter, we will start to bring all the pieces together and show you a step-by-step process of how to take control of your weight, strength, stamina, mental clarity and even a better sex life!

### Step 1 Detoxing:

In this chapter, will be going over the four essential steps to help you do a proper detoxing. They will include the following.

A) Green superfood smoothie fasting

B) Water

C) Hydrotherapy

D) The twist exercise

### A) Green Superfood Smoothies Fasting

Fasting is an ancient custom and is used in almost every religion. From medical history, it has been regarded as one of the most dependable and curative methods to use. You can go to the great historical authorities on medicines such as Socrates, Galleon, Paracelsus and many others who regarded cleansing and fasting as being very beneficial.

Modern physicians have successfully used this method for healing and the treatment of numerous diseases. They have come to the conclusion that many diseases are an accumulation of waste and poisons in the body from improper nutrition and overeating. This overburdens the digestive and assimilative organs while at the same time, slowing up and clogging your system with impurities and poisons. As a result, digestion and elimination become slow, and the functionality of a system is decreased.

> *"Nature's only universal and omnipotent "remedy for healing."*
> — — Dr. Arnold Eherit

By abstaining from solid foods for a time, your bowels, kidneys, skin, and lungs are given the opportunity to rid themselves of an overloaded accumulation of waste in your system, without interference. Fasting is a process of purification that is simple, efficient and quickly shows results. You are helping your body out tremendously by helping it do what it's supposed to do – eliminate toxins, and this can correct any faults that an unhealthy diet or poor life choices have caused. Also, it helps to repair and restore blood and regenerate other tissues of the body. Your doctor may have told you there is no cure for what ails you, or that you must take medication to keep it at bay. This is an ancient healing science of over 2000 years, and you can prove doctors wrong again!

Nearly every disease can be cured, and there is only one remedy.

It's simple – do the opposite of what caused it

The ancient Asian doctors of India, China, and other cultures have made used of fasting for healing for more than 2000 years. They commonly use water with their cleansing activities. Today, we have discovered that liquid vegetable fasting helps to eliminate toxic waste and flood the body with much-needed nutrients which supercharge your body quickly and accelerates healing.

### The Smoothie Myth and the Silver Bullet

Smoothies are all the rage, the big fad and very popular in Hollywood. This liquid diet can be one of the most efficient ways to lose weight and look great. Some vital information you need to know is that most of the smoothies you see for sale in the shopping malls will not help you lose weight. For detox and weight loss purposes, you want smoothies that have no more than 25% fruit. Fruit is a natural sugar, in moderation, it is healthy for you. However, sugar is sugar and drinking very large glasses of natural sugar will not help you lose weight and feel great. Rather, it will most likely give you a spike in your blood sugar, and this is not all that healthy. You want a green leafy smoothie around 75%. We will go over recipes later. The other thing I found highly effective is a 100% all-natural whole super- food. It is the only superfood you can take that will give you growth factors, help tissue repair, has many regenerative properties, fat burning, and anti-aging benefits.

### Benefits:

What if at the end of this fast, you like only to crave delicious foods? What if you looked younger, felt younger, had more stamina and became a better lover? Read on!

### B)  Water

Start your day off with a 16-ounce glass of room temperature water (not cold and no ice) and the juice of one fresh lemon inside. Afterward, drink 16 ounces of water in between smoothies. This is a vital step, as it will help you eliminate and flush out toxins.

**NOTE:** Do you want to feel awful? Between the juicing and the jumping, you will if you don't drink enough water, you will suffer. So drink up!

### C)  Hydrotherapy

> *It takes more than just a good looking body.*
> *You've got to have the heart and soul to go with it*
> - Epictetus

Let me suggest a system of hydrotherapy that is just incredible! How would you like to get the following benefits?

- Stimulate your immune system

- Releases stiffness and relaxes muscles for greater healing
- Deeper sleep
- Better body fluid circulation
- Pumps out toxins
- Weight loss
- Pumps in oxygen
- Refreshes body and mind
- Increased clarity
- Deeper breathing, similar to real exercise
- Feel fantastic, energized and more alive
- More youthful looking skin

Have you ever jumped into a frozen lake, river, or ocean on a hot day? Do you remember how you felt? WOW! What a feeling!

Here's the trick: Shower Hydrotherapy!

It is very simple to do, but it most definitely will be a little challenging for you at first. But, I'm telling you, the rewards are well worth it. Experience this for yourself!

1. 30 to 60 seconds of the hottest water you can take.

2. 30 to 60 seconds of the coldest water you can take.

3. Work your way up to five sets.

4. Always finish with the cold, and attempt to get your entire body wet, even your head.

Ideally, you want to work your way up to 60 seconds, and then five rounds. Remember, always do a couple minutes of cold in the end. Start slowly and work your way up.

If you've never done anything like this, it will be a "BIG SHOCK"!

When I first started doing this, I screamed like a teenager for the first couple days. Gradually, day by day, I increased the length of time until I got up to 60-second mark. Also, you can target areas of your body that are giving you any pain by alternating back and forth with the hot and cold water. This will increase the circulation in those areas, giving you some relief. I have heard of people curing skin cancer with this method. I heard the cancer spot just fell off.

I found this concept many years ago, and to this day, I still use some form of it. My friends think I'm crazy! But the friends who have tried it have felt the benefits.

A six weeks hospital trial showed increases in plasma concentration, T-cell helpers, and lymphocytes. This is an amazing thing to do, and it shows how you have control over making your body heal itself without nutritional supplements or drugs.

Some Swedish families still follow the old tradition today by putting their babies outside for naps in the cold air! What they found is those children are more resistant to disease and sleep deeper!

## D)   The twist

This is simply a twisty motion that you want to do on your rebounder and work your way up to two minutes. It may take you a few days to get up to two minutes however, but this is an activity that helps massage your internal organs, especially your intestines and helps greatly in eliminating toxins. Don't be surprised if your sweat smells bad, it's normal, as soon as you get your body cleansed and eat healthy, you will start to smell sweet.

## Step 2: The ultimate exercise

We are humans, and it's in our nature to move. We were designed to use our bodies to run, jump, play, roll in the grass, pick up and throw things. In our modern sedate world, exercise should be a normal part of your routine. Don't buy some of the modern day guru's hype that you can lose weight without exercise. If you do lose weight, your body will still not be functioning as it was intended. When you exercise, you move around a lot of vital body fluids and hormones. My 35 years of research has brought me to this, and it is what I consider the ultimate exercise. It's fun, easy to do and most of all, you get an incredible benefit with only 10 minutes of a properly done routine.

Would you be interested in an exercise program that takes care of all your needs, which you can do with as little as 10 minutes per day? Some of my favorite activities are swimming and yoga. They have so many benefits to them. However, I find it difficult to get to the pool or ocean frequently, and my yoga discipline takes an hour and a half. These are not so easy to fit into my lifestyle especially with the three-year-old child if you know what I mean? I have done many practices, and I'm absolutely amazed by what I'm going to share with you.

## Jumper

I call it my little jumper, some call it a rebounder, and others call it a mini trampoline. You've seen them around at garage sales on TV info commercials. I used to boo-hoo them, but then I did my research and found they were an effective way to detox and create a healthy exercise program.

I found people curing themselves of cancer and other terminal diseases by jumping! You have more than 75 trillion cells in your body. Your blood system provides oxygen and nutrients, but there is a bigger system than your circulatory system, and it is your lymph system. This has a lot more fluid, but it does not have a pump like your heart. The system functions when you move around when you walk and when you jump. By using a good rebounder and a proper exercise technique, you can pump all 75 trillion cells at one time. My family totally switched our exercise routine, and in the first few months saw tremendous results. My wife at 45 became much more fit, trim and feminine, increasing her breast size. She also noticed a healthier skin, more stamina, and less of a desire to eat junk food. I started to build upper body muscles that were difficult for me before, but now they just happen! I love it! My stamina is up, my clarity of my mind is up, and also, my eyesight is improving, which is a huge bonus.

Some of our close friends also noticed a dramatic increase in our health and immediately ordered their little jumpers.

**WARNING:** Heed my advice, I started off with too many minutes at first, and detox, so much that I ended up in bed for the day! When you get your jumper, you just jump two minutes, and that's all. I would recommend a minimum of two times per day, one in the morning, and another in the evening. If you can do it about four times a day, all the better. Subsequently, you can begin to add on two minutes per time until you get up to 10 minutes. Thousands of folks jump 10 minutes per day and live happy, healthy lives. My wife and I do 10 minutes every morning and evening on an empty stomach before meals, and that serves us well. We are euphoric because our old workout regimen was more than 1 hour.

## The detox move

Do the twist! Just twist at the waist, your feet does not actually come off the mat, you just want to work your way up to two minutes in your 10minute session.

## Oxygenation

Do a gentle bounce with your arms out and elbows bent, with your fingers pointing toward the sky and your mouth open, your elbows can drop down as you jump up and down. Do this for a maximum of one minute, you can start off in 10-second increments. This will help dislodge any junk in your lungs if you cough and spit up, that's a great sign that you are moving the bad boys out of your body. Take it slow until you build up to one minute.

### Not all rebounders and mini - trampolines are the same.

I have bought, tested and tried many brands. It is important that you get a top quality machine. If you get the correct one, you only need to buy it once. I bought an inexpensive jumper, and not only did it feel harsh like it was hurting me, it also fell apart within the first 45 days which makes it very expensive. I've done extensive research, and our family only uses the best. My father taught me to buy the best equipment you can because it's cheaper in the long run. He's correct, our little jumper is awesome and can be used by all, including our three-year-old, as well as our friends who are of a hefty weight. Our little jumper takes it all. There are many great brands out there, do your research. My personal preference is Cellerciser with the balance bar. I find no other quality jumper with this balance bar. This extra bar makes all the difference for working completely different muscle groups, and in addition to building firm butt and stomach muscles, it also works on all kinds of skin tone and eliminates double chins. We travel a lot, and also invested in the folding one with its case. The link at the back of the book will give you a $40 bonus that includes some helpful books, videos and such. Cellerciser information is very thorough, just follow through their start up plan as directed, and double their daily routine for your detox program.

In my family, this little piece of equipment has replaced our yoga routine, one-hour bike ride and weights. Now, when we do those things, it's just for fun, and it's a bonus.

*The little jumper is true inexpensive health insurance.*

## Five-minute Temporary alternative workout:

If, for whatever reason, you do not have access to a jumper, you will need some form of exercise to keep things moving. If you have a program you're doing already, that's great, stick with it. If not, follow the program below twice a day, once in the morning, and once in the evening. To start with, you may have to do each exercise only 15 to 30 seconds working your way up to the full minute.

## Five-minute workout

1. One-minute jumping jacks
2. One-minute push-ups
3. One-minute Squats (hands behind your head)
4. One-minute jumping jacks
5. One-minute walking

Would you like to do the ultimate workout in just 10 minutes per day? Then it's a must for you put this high-quality jumper on your wish list. This one piece of equipment can replace all your other workout machines, practices, and trips to classes and gyms.

## Step 3

## Inducing the relaxation response

On the subject of anti-aging, all the activities in this chapter will help to reverse aging. Anything that you can do to help you will also improve your appearance and roll the clock back. I believe the number one thing you can do is meditation/prayer/quiet time. Find your way to do it that works for you. For me, it's like bookends. I start my day with 15 minutes, throw in a few minutes of thankfulness, and I repeat it just before I lay my head down for the night. My bookends!

Enjoy

Some call it meditation; some call it prayer. It's a form of focusing, a way to quiet the mind, to be thankful for what you have and focus on where you want to be.

From the Washington Times – Aug 14, 2003

*A new study shows [that] people who underwent meditation training produced more antibodies to a flu vaccine than people who did not meditate. Those who took part in the meditation study also showed signs of increased activity in areas of the brain related to positive emotion, as compared to people who did not meditate.*

CBS News – Aug 27, 2003

*People who meditate these days come from all walks of life and aren't necessarily weird New Agers or pretentious actors. Students, lawyers, West Point cadets, athletes, prisoners, and government officials all meditate. It's supposed to help depression, control pain, increase longevity, slow down cancers, invigorate the immune system, and significantly reduce blood pressure. Time magazine recently reported that "meditation can sometimes be used to replace Viagra."*

Time Magazine – Aug 4, 2003

*Not only do studies show that meditation boosts the immune system, but brain scans also suggest that it may be rewiring the brains to reduce stress. It's recommended by more and more physicians as a way to prevent, slow or at least control the pain of chronic diseases like heart conditions, AIDS, cancer and infertility.*

**"Inducing the Relaxation Response."**

Inducing the Relaxation Response is a phrase coined by Dr. Herbert Benson. He is a researcher that discovered that in only eight weeks of meditation, committing to 15 minutes per day; you can literally change your DNA structure!

Meditation is not a religion, and I am in no way suggesting a different spiritual belief or religious following. This is just what actually works for me after many years of trying different things.

**Here's a short list of just some of the many benefits:**

- Increased health
- Increased happiness
- More control, thinking more clearly
- Less stress, more energy
- Better eating habits
- Increased calm and serenity
- Weight loss
- Stronger immune system

**WOW!** Meditation is a great thing. There are hundreds of books on meditation, and I have studied many. I have even gone as far as taking a tenday, vegetarian, no talking, 6 hours per day meditation retreat. I'm not suggesting that you need to do that; however, what I will suggest is a very simple, easy to do meditation program that you can learn in a few minutes.

A few minutes of meditation, every day can change your life! It certainly has changed mine.

*I believe it is the number one self-improvement thing that you can do for yourself, PERIOD!*

~Marcus Norman

Actual meditation is very simple. Find a safe, quiet, private place for yourself. Don't worry about being in a full lotus yoga position, just sit comfortably. I sit on a soft rug on my heels, my hands in my lap, my back and shoulders arched back a little bit. You don't want to be slouched over or leaning. A good posture is one when you look dignified, sitting like a king or queen when you are relaxed and self-confident.

1.          You will want to anchor yourself, just like a boat on the shore. Just something to keep you tethered and focused. I have found a very simple way to do this, close your eyes, focus on your breathing, follow the breath going in your nostrils and into your lungs - seeing the number 1 tumbling as it goes into your nostril,  then follow the number 1 as it exhales, leaving your lungs and nostrils.

2.          Repeat this sequence as you count up.

Okay, simple enough right? Yeah, it's true, it sounds simple enough. However, what you may find is that your mind wanders, and you lose track of the numbers - that is very normal. I would be very surprised if you could just count to 10 without losing track. Just refocus on counting and the breath.

Here is a little trick I found to be very helpful. On Day 1, I just meditated for 60 seconds. That's it! Just 60 seconds, 1 minute only. Everybody can do that. Then on Day 2, I meditated for only 2 minutes. The same goes for Day 3 - I meditated for only 3 minutes, and this pattern continued day after day. Okay, just work your way up to 15 minutes per day. Although it depends on how quickly you breathe, ideally, counting to 50 should be about 15 minutes. However, for some that can be as much as 75 breaths. Maximum meditation results are when you breathe deep and slow, without any sound on the inhale and exhale. You can even go for the expert level by putting a little pause at the end of your inhale and exhale. When you meditate 15 minutes per day, for 30 days, you will see vast changes in your life. What I found was a huge change in my emotional state. I was calmer and more relaxed, and I also focused much better. Personally, I do 15 minutes the very first thing in the morning, and then I do 15 minutes the very last thing just before I go to sleep. This is an excellent way to create an extraordinary day!

At one time in my life, I was meditating 3 hours a day! Wow! Okay, another little secret, 15 minutes a day of quality mediation is all you need. It seemed to me that things happened in my life much easier, the stuff that I wanted, or things I wanted to happen just happened with little or no effort on my part.

Enjoy! Your life will never be the same!

*"Eight weeks of meditation - 15 minutes per day- can literally change your DNA structure!"*

\- Dr. Herbert Benson

# Chapter 5

## I Don't Believe in Supplements

Do you believe in supplements? At one time in my life, I was on more than $600 per month of healthy nutritional supplements. The issue I found about taking supplements is that scientists discovered some excellent component like a vitamin or mineral, or some nutrient that can enhance our life experience. My belief is that nature has created the perfect whole foods for us. All of the vitamins, minerals and nutrients we need are included in them and all the things that make them bio-available for our bodies. So, when modern scientists separate what they see as important, it usually is not being delivered with all the other components that nature had intended to help them quickly assimilate into our bodies and be fully absorbed. Some supplements have actually healed or cured people of many challenging diseases. However, they must be taken with caution because some can have an adverse long-term effect. Nutritional supplements have their appropriate time and place.

I found it better to spend your resources on healthy foods and proper exercises. This is a better method that ensures the delivery of to your body, all the vitamins and minerals that you need in the natural delivery system; that's in balance and much more available for your body.

Sometimes nutritional supplements are used to support the healing process in patients. But note, for example, if a health practitioner is giving high doses of vitamin C to help correct an ailment. He will also have the patient eat foods that are high in vitamin C, as these foods with all its other components and micronutrient nutrients are what will help deliver the manufactured vitamin C. Does that make sense?

I no longer take massive amounts of nutritional supplements. In fact, I take no supplement. There is, however, one thing I take, and I give it to my whole family. It's not a supplement; it is a superfood. It's a complete superfood. It comes from the very first liquid that sets up the immune system in mammals, the very first food we were ever given to set up our immune system. It's called colostrum, and colostrum is life-giving and without it, mammals would just die. The kind I use is called bovine colostrum and it comes from cows. It is the pre-milk that comes before the actual milk for the calf.

This bovine colostrum, I find helps tremendously with this smoothie fasting diet. It cuts down on inflammation and helps to heal the intestinal track. It is an immune system booster.

It is best to use a bovine colostrum powder that has the following characteristics. It's important to note not all colostrums are the same. Some are collected on the 2nd ,3rd or 4th days and have significantly reduced beneficial properties while others are highly processed which makes them cheaper, but, however, a lot less helpful to you.

**Recommended Specifications:**

- First milking (Procured within the first 24 hours).

- Low-temperature, rapid processing for maximum bioavailability.

- At least 18% PRp's peptides immunoglobulins (You don't want the 40% immunoglobulins because they are more processed, and not in a natural balance for delivery).

- The farmer is certified for being pesticide, hormone and antibiotic free.

For myself and my patience, I use BodyBoost in capsules and powder form. You're going to want to use powder for your detox program. Inner harmony LLC brought this product to the market nearly 18 years ago; they were one of the very first companies to lead the way and bring a cost-effective superfood to the masses. Before that, it was just used in small batches to heal people of terminal diseases, major health issues or those who knew about it or could afford it. There is a lot more information about Colostrum and an excellent transcript of a doctor's radio broadcast at their website http://colostrumbodyboost.com/. The bonus is you no longer have to buy it in the health food store and can buy it from Amazon directly, with free shipping that is more than 50% discount from the health food store.

TEN-DAY GREEN SUPERFOOD SMOOTHIE CLEANSE

## Step 5: Smoothies

Your Green Superfood Smoothie Diet Plan

Smoothie template to create five smoothies for the day.

2 cups of water (adjust amount as needed to help it liquefy)

Oil = can be 1 tablespoon of coconut oil, fish oil or nuts and seeds, walnuts, almonds, cashews, sesame seeds, etc.

25% fruit = apples and berries, etc.

75% green leafy vegetables = spinach, kale, mixed baby greens, etc.

4 tablespoons of 100% whole bovine colostrum powder (after cleanse, just 1tbs per 16oz smoothie)

2 tablespoons of vegetable protein, hemp, pea powder (protein = no hunger)

Generally, you want to pick just one from each of the following categories below. Some basic rules are:

1.     Make use of fresh ingredients as much as possible, frozen is okay. However, NO canned, bottled or preserved foods.

2.     No dairy

3.     No dairy like substances, like almond or soy milk (they are highly processed and have sugar)

4.     Very little to no sweeteners

5.     About 2 cups fruit to 4 cups of packed greens and 1 cup of water

## Liquid base:

1 cup of water

1 cup of green tea

1 cup of your favorite healthy tea

## Healthy oils:

Pick one per recipe. Organic, nuts must be raw, and oils must be cold pressed.

2 tablespoon of coconut oil

2 tablespoons flaxseed oil

A quarter cup of raw cashews

One and half and avocado

2 tablespoons of flaxseed (sprouted is even much better)

2 tablespoons of Chia seed (sprouted is even much better)

**Fruits:**

It is best to keep fruits to a maximum percentage of 25% of the ingredients. Feel free to vary the amount according to the recipe, the amount listed below are just suggestions.

One Apple with skin

Half of a banana

One-quarter of a peeled orange

One-quarter of a lime

One-quarter of a lemon

One-quarter of a pineapple

Grapefruit

Blueberries

Pomegranates

Raspberries

Pears with the skin

Oranges

Kiwi

Cantaloupe

Apricots Veggies:

Brussels sprouts

Cauliflower

Bok choy

Beets

Pumpkin

Kale

Broccoli

Celery

Cucumber with the skin

All leafy greens, for example, Arugula, Spinach, and Baby Kale.

Collard greens

Spring greens

Swiss chard

Green cabbage

Arugula

Barley grass

Sprouts

Dandelion greens

Mustard greens

Mint (use in smaller quantities)

Parsley (use in smaller quantities)

Cilantro (coriander)

Mixed baby leaf salad mix

Carrots (small amounts and not during cleanse)

Tomatoes

## TEN-DAY GREEN SUPERFOOD SMOOTHIE CLEANSE

**Super foods**: always put in colostrum and one of the following

1 teaspoon colostrum per 16oz smoothie

Kale

¼ teaspoon of Camu Camu

Maca

Wheat grass

Avocados

Hemp protein powder

2 tablespoons of raw cocoa powder or nibs

2 tablespoons of Chia seeds

2 tablespoons of coconut oil

1/8 teaspoon to half a teaspoon of cayenne pepper (adjust to tolerance level of heat)

Goji beans

**Nuts:**

5 to 10 raw almonds (soak overnight)

5 to 10 raw walnuts (soak overnight)

5 to 10 raw cashew nuts (soaked overnight)

**Protein powders:**

Pea protein powder

Hemp powder

Rice powder

**Sweeteners:**

Try to use zero or no sweeteners, but I do understand if at first, you need a little to make it more palatable and that's okay.

**Other Ingredients:**

Mesquite Powder

Cayenne pepper dry
Medical mushrooms

This is your basic detox smoothie cleanse template. After the cleanse, you can vary the amounts of the ingredients, for example, add more fruit at subtraction or substitute ingredients. Note that in the back of the book, there are over 100 recipes and content suggestions

You're going to want to drink about 5 per day, in about 16 ounces each. Please take them when you want, however, an example of a schedule might be:

6 AM, 9 AM, 12 PM, 3 PM, 6 PM.

I make them all up at one time and put them in airtight glass containers. That way, they stay for the day and are easy to access.

**Five-step summary**

Fasting detoxes are more than 2000 years old and have been used by hundreds of thousands of people throughout history to heal ailments. The modern version uses nutrition rich vegetable smoothies to accelerate the healing process of your body. Proper exercise assists you in removing toxic waste and enhances your mental state and your overall well-being. Meditation can be the number one self-improvement thing you can do for yourself beyond anything else in this book. If you're happy, it goes a long way in helping yourself and others. You don't need a lot of nutritional supplements if you eat healthily. Green superfood detoxing smoothies will flush out your system and flood your body with needed nutrients and reset your body clock so you can crave healthy foods and stop the junk food addiction cycle.

In the next chapter, we will be going over what people ate 250,000 years ago, and why it is important for you to know. It may not be what you think.

# Chapter 6

## 250,000 Years of Proof

# A Dietary Habit of Over 250, 000 Years
# A Healing Modality of 2,000 Years

Some resources will show you that 250,000 years ago, we were huntergatherers. If you dive into it deeper, you will see some of the studies are based on what they found around ancient fire pits that were mostly bones. I guess dried corn husks and apple cores didn't make it to the 250,000 years journey. Further studies have revealed that men lived mainly on grains, fresh vegetables, and fruit.

> *"All large verifiable human populations in history were fit and trim*
> *and the bulk of the calories came from starch, vegetables and fruit*
> *without exception"*
>
> — — Dr. John McDougall

Once you finish this detox program, we will go over the details of an all you can eat diet plan and be healthy fit and trim, doesn't that sound great!?

> *Research shows that a diet consisting of whole grains, healthy*
> *starches, vegetables and fruit*

Have no weight issues 100% of the time!

**The 2000 year history of Asian doctors**

Asian doctors in India, China, and other areas have employed fasting to heal their patients and to correct maladies for more than 2000 years.

*"Fasting is highly beneficial in practically all kinds of stomach and intestinal disorders and in serious conditions of the kidneys and liver. It is a miracle cure for diseases and offers the only hope of permanent cure in many cases."*

~ Dr. S. R. Jindal

Dr. Max Gerson started healing people with cancer in the 1930s. He discovered that a diet consisting mostly of fresh vegetables juice, fresh vegetables, fruits and whole grains reduced, if not eliminated many illnesses, some of them being terminal! There are many clinics based on his research around the world that cure people every day of incurable diseases!

*The doctors of the future will no longer treat the human frame with drugs, but rather will cure and prevent disease with nutrition.*

−− Thomas Edison

# Chapter 7

## Weight Loss Motivation

### Dr. George Sets You up to Succeed

In this chapter, we are going to go over how Dr. George will set you up to be successful with this weight loss program. Because, most of us have been eating a Standard American Diet. A very helpful and a much easier transition into the ten-day superfood smoothie cleanse will be provided with the pointers in this chapter.

At the age of 24, I had the rude awakening that I had contracted genital herpes. I was in a tremendous amount of pain, not only from the outbreak in my groins, but also emotionally. How was I ever going to attract an excellent mate to marry? Who would want to be with me? Maybe I should just end it now? The Doctor gave me a list of medications I should be taking, but after I had done my research, I understood that they would not eliminate my herpes symptoms. I was told it was incurable, and there would be side effects to my health from taking this medication long-term. I cured myself with the basic concept in this book. Pay close attention to setting yourself up to be successful for the ten-day cleanse, as it will help you transition into it. And if you're like me and have played hard with your body and put it away wet, I'm here to say not only am I symptom-free and live a happy, healthy life, I have also attracted the most amazing woman into my life with one of the results being our little Angel of a daughter! Life is good!

One week before you start the ten-day smoothie cleanse, you will want to make some dietary changes. Start reducing the following, and by the end of the week, they should be totally out of your diet, just in time for you to start the cleanse.

Stimulants = coffee, alcohol, and chocolate

Animal protein = beef, chicken, seafood

Valueless carbohydrates = donuts, pastries and other junk foods

Tobacco = chewing tobacco or cigarettes ( This is a big subject, you understand it's not part of a healthy lifestyle, it's your choice)

**Things to start right away that will help you out:**

- Order your colostrum in powder form

- Order your jumper, the one with the balance bar

- Until your little jumper shows up, start exercising morning and evening, a 15-minute walk is just fine. Please note that if you have not been previously doing any exercise, it is better just to start with two minutes per time and add two minutes on per day. That will make it much easier to be to get going.

- Start doing the hydrotherapy today! As soon as you finish this book get yourself in the shower!

**Transition off the cleanse:**

It is crucial when you transition off of a fast like this. You have been flooding your body with nutrients, and also removing massive amounts of toxins. You will be feeling amazing, an on-top-of-the-world type of feeling, it is, however, imperative that you transition back to healthy, more traditional solid foods. Some folks get excited because of their results on a liquid diet. However, I would only recommend a maximum of 21 days on a liquid diet like this. After your detox, here are the transition steps I recommend. It's possible to undo all the excellent benefits you've gained by going back to poor food choices and the binging of certain types of foods right after the cleanse. It is very easy for your weight gain to come back if you don't transition and change your diet to serve you better.

Day 11- create your smoothies for the day except exchange two smoothies for one meal of salad and a clean protein.

Day 12- have two light, clean meals and to smoothies

Day 13- three light meals, salad based with some pure protein, nothing heavy

Day 14- all-you-can-eat from your new healthy diet list below

## All-you-can-eat healthy diet

Animal pathogens such as salmonella or E. coli are easily transferred to humans. However, in the vegetable world, if a vegetable gets sick, we cannot get their sickness.

TEN-DAY GREEN SUPERFOOD SMOOTHIE CLEANSE

Animal products are on the top of the food chain, which means that they can have many levels of toxic chemicals like DDT, pesticides and artificial fertilizers in them. When we ingest them, they can become highly concentrated. One simple example that these chemicals have reached our oceans is the fact that eating tuna today has a risk of having mercury in it. The simple solution is plant-based foods, they are low on the food chain, clean plant-based proteins and have a little to no chemical buildup in them.

## Protein Myth

You never have to think if you are eating enough protein. Marketing has convinced us that if we don't eat massive quantities of meat, we will not have enough protein to survive. I take this opportunity again to remind you of the fact that for all large verifiable human populations in history, the bulk of their calories came from vegetables, starch and fruits. These people were fit, trim and healthy without exception. Some of the top athletes in the world live on raw food that does not include any animal protein.

## Here is your easy stay on diet

Some studies have shown 88% retention after one year on this diet, which is a surprising statistic because most people give up diets in a few weeks.

What's different about this diet? It's all you can eat, it's satisfying and leaves no hungry feeling.

## Things to abstain from:

Animal proteins: they turn on the cancer-causing program in your body

No dairy or meat

No processed oils

No highly processed foods

No foods containing corn syrup or artificial sweeteners

## Foods to eat:

Oils: get your oil from eating nuts (walnuts, almonds, sunflower seeds), fruits and vegetables (avocados),

Carbohydrates: you want clean carbohydrates, for example, brown rice, beans, table corn, whole-grain flours, etc. Organic fruits and vegetables.

**Tip:** I went to my kitchen cabinets, freezer, and refrigerator and gave away the so-called foods or the things that I thought were food. Believe me, it's helpful if you have a weak moment. If you have to live with other people who must have their Oreo cookies, tell them you can't be trusted and they need to hide them from you! Ha ha!

## Be active

What do you like to do? You need to move your body because you're human. Sign up for a sports team, go dancing, bowl, row the boat across the lake. Pick something fun that you like to do that will get you involved.

It is important to start a week in advance in order to cut out the major groups of stimulants like coffee, alcohol, and chocolate. Stop smoking, cut out any junk food such as valueless carbs like pastries and sugary stuff. It will make it much easier to do the detox.

Start exercising, make sure to order your colostrum and your jumper ahead of time so it will be there before you're ready to start your ten-day program. You can start your hydrotherapy today. After the detox, remember to transition slowly into your new healthy lifestyle diet. Go to your kitchen and throw out or donate all of the food that doesn't fit your new lifestyle, and start some fun activity that will keep your body moving always.

Now, let's continue to the frequently asked questions in the next chapter.

*Most of you do not believe that it is your natural state of being to be well.*

*– – Abraham*

# Chapter 8

## F.A.Q.

**Q: *Can I do a green smoothie detox program if I'm diabetic?***

A: Yes! Countless people I know have received tremendous benefits, even to the point of not having to take the medication any longer. Keep an eye on how you feel, and make sure you do not go over that 25% fruit limit in your smoothies.

**Q: *Are my medications toxic?***

A: To get an idea of how toxic your medication is in the long and short-term. The degrading health ramifications these drugs can play in your health, read the enclosed warning pamphlet that should be with your prescription medications.

**Q: *What do I do if I generally drink alcohol?***

A: Start reducing your alcohol intake a week or two in advance of the actual detox cleanse and reduce your consumption down to zero before you start the cleanse.

**Q: *What if I find it too challenging for me?***

A: If you've never done anything like this before, for some people it may be too much. Adjust the detox diet so you can do some part of it. Take one or two weeks before the detox part of the cleanse, and slowly remove any stimulants (coffee, alcohol, and chocolate). Start weaning yourself off of junk food, valueless carbs and sugary foods like pastries. Start drinking the recommended water amount, start walking two minutes per day twice a day, and then increase it by two-minute increments until you get to 15 minutes. If you need further help during the detox, you can replace two smoothies with a light meal of salad and a clean protein. Don't beat yourself up, the main point is to move forward. Do what you can for now, even though you may not lose 10 pounds in the ten-day cleanse, however, you will be resetting your body clock that will help you move on to a healthier diet. Think long-term, no yo-yo dieting effects. Once you start, you can lose a little bit of weight every week that stays off. How would you feel if you lost 1 pound every week and it stayed off?

Q: *What if I take medication?*

A: I cannot give you medical advice in this book without physically seeing you. You should seek your local medical adviser. Note, many people who go on to the start have reduced or eliminated their medications. Please, keep in mind it's a case-by-case situation.

Q: *My standard blender is making chunkies and not smoothies what do I do?*

A: Smoothie blenders such as the Vitamix, Blendtec, and the Bullet are designed to make smoothies. Household blenders, however, can be adequate for this ten-day cleanse. The trick is to put the liquid in first and then adequate amounts. You may need to put a little extra water, and then put in half the ingredients, after which you should turn off the blender once it is nice and smooth to retain the balance. Try to keep it all less than 60 seconds for best nutrition results.

Q: *What if I take supplements?*

A: This is a good time to stop your supplements, as this will help flush out your system and give you a fresh start. Then after that, if you think you need them, you can continue. However in my household, we put our efforts more toward healthier foods and not supplements.

Q: *Can I gain weight on superfood green smoothie diet?*

A: It's difficult to gain weight if you do it properly. However, if you do no exercise and drink mostly fruit smoothies, you can gain unhealthy weight.

Q: *Does blending destroy nutrients?*

A: Any processing of foods destroys nutrients. It is recommended that you use a blender for less than one minute when creating smoothies.

Q: *Is a green smoothie detox program okay for people with Candida?*

A: Many Candida sufferers have experienced an elimination of their condition. Monitor yourself carefully, exchange other fruits for oranges, grapefruits, lemons, and limes. Also contact your healthcare professional.

**Q: Do I exercise during a detox?**

A: It's a good idea while you're detoxing to move your body. That said, keep in mind that if you feel bad and it's very uncomfortable, stop or reduce

the amount you're doing. Try sticking with the regimented recommended amounts in this book. In the long run, you always want to do exercise for a healthy happy body. Don't listen to some gurus telling you that you can create your proper healthy weight without exercise, that is just unnatural and baloney.

**Q: What if I want to eat solid foods?**

A: If you eat solid foods during the detox, it puts a different demand on your digestive system. The liquefied foods that you are creating with smoothies are easy to digest; hence, it gives your digestive system a break so that energy can go into cleaning and healing you. So, when you throw in solid foods into the mix, it's not as effective. There are some popular books out there that have you snacking in between smoothies. This is not the most effective way to do a cleanse; it's just their way to keep you from being hungry. The trick to not being hungry is to drink 5 X 16-ounce smoothies with protein powder. The protein powder curbs your hunger. Also, drink 16 ounces of water in between the smoothies and do your exercises. Once you get started, you will not feel hungry. If it's still an issue for some, you can add in cayenne pepper, as it will spice up your smoothies. This, however, is not for everyone, but personally, I love it.

**Q: How often should I have a bowel movement during the cleanse?**

A: At first, the frequency may be more than normal, and they may be loose even to the point of diarrhea. Remember your body is dumping toxins, after a few days you will be mostly urinating due to the high volume of liquids and no real solid foods.

**Q: How long can I do the superfood green smoothies detox program?**

A: I would not recommend doing this program for more than 21 days. You can drink them indefinitely as long as you put in at least one healthy meal per day. If you do that, it's possible to keep losing 1 pound per week depending on your situation.

**Q: Will it affect my sleep?**

A: It's possible that you will experience variations in your sleep pattern. Once you get through the first few days, you will have a lot more energy. You may even feel like you don't need so much sleep, but I highly recommend that you sleep as much as you can, as this allows your body to use the energy for healing.

Q: *Is detoxing painful?*

A: There may be a day or two where you are uncomfortable, feeling headaches, diarrhea, achy body and you want to sleep all day. It is imperative that you remember that this will pass and stay on the regimen. Some people even find that they can sleep a whole day if you're one of them, by all means do it as your body is healing.

Q: *Is a liquid diet a fast way to lose weight?*

A: A liquid diet is one of the fastest ways to lose weight! That said, you must be very careful because if you jump back into your regular eating routine, you will just get back to the weight you were before, or worse, gain even more weight. This is the effect of a yo-yo diet, and that's why it is so important for you to follow the last four days as recommended in this book. After this, switch to an all-you-can-eat healthy diet that is also described in detail in this book. This will take you off the yo-yo diet effect, and start you on your journey of a healthy, happy and energized life.

Q: *Is this a low-carb diet?*

A: No, it's filled with quality carbohydrates. A fresh, whole ripe fruit which is an excellent source of vitamins, minerals and antioxidants also includes lots of fiber. This is not to be confused with bad carbs that we all know are not so healthy, like donuts, pasta, white rice, white breads, sodas, valueless carbs, sweetened beverages and sweetened baked goods. These types of foods are the leaders in the obesity epidemic in the world today. Having stated this, while a detox cleanse, you still want to limit your intake of calories. Any consumption of excess calories can be a reason for weight gain. Stick to the plan during the detox phase, it will set up your body not to crave the bad carbs. Subsequently, we will show you how to eat all you can with your new healthy diet.

Q: *What if I'm a smoker?*

A: My father smoked for 35 years! Once he quit, he could never look back, owing to his amazement at how much better he felt. Nonetheless, one side effect was weight gain, and once he started drinking proper amounts of water and adjusted his diet, it was no longer an issue. If you're smoker, the choice is up to you. But then again, you know the truth; you know that smoking does not serve your health interests.

TEN-DAY GREEN SUPERFOOD SMOOTHIE CLEANSE

### Q: Juice fasting or smoothie fasting which is better?

A: They both have their benefits. The additional benefits of smoothie cleansing is that it has fiber, and when you add protein powder; it helps you feel satisfied and not hungry. They are also much quicker and easier to make, especially when you're creating superfood smoothies.

### Q: Can I just live on superfood green smoothies and not eat food?

A: A superfood green smoothie ten-day diet plan is temporary. It has three purposes; the first one is to rid your body of built-up toxins. The second one is to give you lots of nutritional support while you're going through this healing process. The Third, and this is a big one, is to reset your body clock not to crave junk food. After you've done the ten-day program, you can always keep in one or two green smoothies in a day, and this can create a continual weight loss atmosphere until you reach your ideal weight.

### Q: Is it safe?

A: Please, consult your healthcare professional, especially for a diabetic. Tens of thousands of people have done this type of cleanse, but it's still crucial that you realize it's a case-by-case basis. There are many factors to be considered, your health at this moment, the medication you are on and so on. That said, we have found no real issues with it being unsafe. A few people have stopped or cut the program back and turned to their needs because they did not feel well. Most likely, they had very toxic body systems. After the second or third day, most people will feel like they've never felt before in their lives, clearheaded, energized, and full of life.

### Q: How long do the smoothies last?

A: If you put the smoothie in an airtight container, preferably glass and keep it cool, they should be usable for up to 24 hours. Keeping in mind that the sooner you drink it, the better as the nutritional value drops as time goes on.

**Did You Know You Could Find Happiness in the Produce Aisle?**

*We know fruits and vegetables are good for our bodies, but a recent study of nearly 14,000 people suggests they could help our mental health too. About 33% of those who scored high in mental well-being reported digging into five or more portions of produce a day, compared to just fewer than 7% who ate less than one. Fruits and veggie eaters may have other healthy habits, so many factors could be at play, says Sverio Strangers, Ph.D., M.D., a study co-author. It is also a theory that certain antioxidants and produce may influence our levels of optimism.*

This is an excerpt from
Dr. Oz's
"THE GOOD LIFE" Magazine
January/February 2015 edition.

# Chapter 9

## Dr. George's and Marcus's Success Tips and Tricks

The following are some things we observed in the process of helping people through this life-changing experience:

**Chew**: The first mouthful of smoothie, take your time and chew it. This starts to set up your digestive system. Take as long as you can, the digestive juices in your mouth will come out and also signal to your stomach what's coming. This is no race, and gulping down 16 ounces of veggies will not be as much benefit to you, better to take it slow and steady.

**Hungry feeling:** Protein powder goes a long way in curbing that feeling. After the first few days, you should not feel hungry. Also, keep in mind that between the smoothies and the water intake about every hour and a half, you're putting in 16 ounces of fluid in your system. That should keep your belly full, and your satisfaction needs to be met. If you however still feel a little hungry, you can put one teaspoon of sea salt (Himalayan is my preference) in your next few smoothies. Just know it will pass, go for a walk, breathe, have water or tea, talk with a friend, and create a distraction.

**Blenders:** If you have a Vitamix, Blendtec, or Bullet, you should have no issues with mixing. Regular household blenders will also work, but when using these, make sure you have adequate fluid or water, and always put that in first and you may have to put in half the solid ingredients in at first then the rest once it gets going. There's a benefit to having one of the heavy duty ones like the Vitamix because you can mix all five drinks at the same time. Smaller blenders, you'll have to make two batches, which is also fine, as it can give you two different flavors if you so, please.

**Weight fluctuation:** Do not get on the scale every day, your weight will go up and down, and you don't want to make yourself crazy do you? My recommendation is to weigh yourself the week before, weigh yourself the day of the detox program, weigh yourself on day five, and at the end of the program. Then after that, you may check your weight once a week or less.

**Can I put ice in my drinks?** I know it sounds good to have a cold smoothie. Nevertheless, we're following a detox program and cold drinks, especially ice can cool down the digestive system, and we do not want to impair any digestive processes at this point. After the cleanse, feel free to make yourself a nice fruit smoothie with honey and coconut cream, yummy! However, on a needed basis, it's best not to drink anything cool.

**Does it taste good?** If it does, it's a bonus. The drinks are designed to do their job and do a detox. If you need to make it more palatable for yourself, look at the ingredients and see how you can change them. For example, you could add a little maple syrup or a little bit of more fruit. Keeping in mind that you want to keep the sugar down because that's what is optimal for detoxing.

**Water:** If you do not drink a lot of water right now, start the week before. You will most likely start detoxing just from the water intake alone. So, if you feel a little off, tired and cranky, it would be normal. Get your rest and keep hydrating.

**Herbal teas:** They can be used in place of water in smoothies, you can also drink green teas and detox teas.

**Diabetics:** People who suffer from diabetes mellitus stand to gain a lot in this program. In spite of this, it is essential that you are very mindful of what's going on with you and your body. Seek professional help immediately if you're having issues beyond what is described in this detox program. Note that it's normal to feel poor, tired, smell bad, have diarrhea for up to a few days.

**Constipation:** With all these fluids going in, normally this is not an issue. However, if you find yourself stopped up, mix a half teaspoon of sea salt and 8 ounces of warm water, then drink two more 8-ounce glasses of warm water. The next step is to stay near the toilet because it will be calling.

**Curbing your appetite:** Jump or exercise about 20 minutes before you eat, it will set up your body not to consume so much food. This is a great hack, test it out for yourself.

**Toxins:** Creams, lotions, potions, makeup, hair and nails products. If you won't put it in your mouth, don't put it on your skin.

TEN-DAY GREEN SUPERFOOD SMOOTHIE CLEANSE

After the detox program, stop eating a minimum of 3 hours before you sleep.

Go for a walk after a meal. People who do weigh 12% less than the average population.

Spend your time and money on improving your health and well-being, and not paying medical bills and expensive drugs which only poisons you in the long run.

**Soak your nuts:** by soaking nuts you start the sprouting process, this begins to release latent energy. Some of the food benefits can be multiple times more than dried nuts. Overnight is good 24 hours is even better. Nuts have phytic acid. Phytic acid is also found in grains and legumes. Just as with grains and legumes, soaking nuts is essential for proper digestions. When eating nuts that haven't been soaked, the phytic acid binds to minerals in the gastrointestinal tract and cannot be absorbed in the intestine and too many bound minerals can lead to mineral deficiencies. By soaking, you are breaking down the phytic acid so it can be absorbed properly.

Nuts also have high amounts of enzymes inhibitors. Another reason unsoaked nuts are hard to digest. Soaking nuts neutralizes the enzymes allowing for proper digestion. Reduces cravings, and beneficial for weight loss.

**Keep it to yourself:** When I'm doing any self-improvement work, I find it best to keep it to myself. I don't tell anybody, and there is a big reason for that. Unfortunately, most people do not want to improve themselves, and especially do not want to see other people improve themselves. As a result, they may not be supportive, or they may call you crazy. Another reason is, say, for example, you only lose 4 pounds and not 10; your friends will get on you and say yeah, look, it didn't work. But if you tell them nothing, and they see that you lost 4 pounds, you are trimmed up, have better energy, focus, and your stamina is increased, they know something's up. Just maybe they'll have kind words of congratulations, and the net result is you move forward in the direction you want to go.

Is there a "Fountain of Youth" potion? Turn to the next chapter to find out.

Vamanos!

# Chapter 10

## Anti-aging, Fountain of youth and Polyproline-Rich Peptides

**What If You Could Reverse the Clock?**

**Exercise and anti-aging:**

When you use, you turn on the front part of your brain called the prefrontal cortex. This is the CEO of your brain, as it creates neurotransmitters. Brain-derived neurotrophic factors are like miracle growths for your brain; they keep your cells young and perky. Exercise is one of the best ways to stop any cognitive decline, for example, Alzheimer's. You want to keep the brain plastic and allow it to grow with new information. Examples of ways to do that can be to go study a new language, instrument or a new subject.

*"Your body is a temple, but only if you treat it as one."*

--Astrid Alauda

**Whole Superfood:**

One of the most notable medical journals in the world is the "New England Journal of Medicine". It stated that the most effective way to stop or slow down the aging process is to replace the hormonal factors that are the cause of healthy cellular structures in the body. After the age of 20, the levels of growth hormones in our bodies are reduced considerably, with time, our body start to lose elasticity of the skin and muscle tone that causes sagging and wrinkles. Bone mass can be reduced, and our feet, nose, hands and ears can get larger. Isolated hormone replacement therapy synthesized from plants is not an identical match for the hormones in the human body. The side effects can be life-threatening.

I tried human growth hormones, the results were every month, I needed more and more. I started to feel concerned about any possible side effects, so

I switched to peptide whole foods. I take no supplements, only this whole superfood.

That whole superfood is colostrum, and it's a perfect balance of immune and growth factors. In the clinical trials of its subjects, it had safely increased the lgF-1 to pre-puberty levels. The net result is an increase in muscle weight and strength. When you add in the GH from the colostrum, it is also shown to tone the muscles, return elasticity to the skin, increase bone density and melt away the body fat. Could this be the fountain of youth superfood?

> *Advanced age is associated with reduced levels of growth hormones:*
> *GH and IgF — 1. Induction of GH and IgF — 1 increases body*
> *weight to muscle growth of age subjects.*
> Doctors Ulmen, Sommerland and Kottner, Department of pathology
> and pharmacology, --University of Gothenburg, Sahlgren hospital
> Stockholm, Sweden

The RNA is an active intelligence part of a DNA that can help to produce the proteins needed to repair and build up the body.

Youth and aging researcher, Dr. Benjamin Frank showed that the RNA is one of the most critical anti-aging factors. LgF — 1 which occurs naturally in colostrum is the **only substance known to stimulate the growth and the repair of key nucleic acids, DNA and RNA.**

Colostrum helps maintain blood glucose levels to help serve the brain. GF and LgF-1 are some of the smallest particles known to have crossed the blood-brain barrier, and the net result is that they assist tremendously with nerve synapses in the brain. In turn enhances your mental acuity, increases serotonin levels and has the side effect of brightening your moods. This might be an important reason alone for you to want to take this superfood.

> *Do you know that colostrum repairs your body's essential*
> *DNA and RNA?*
> ~Dr. Keech

The aging process is a depletion of our natural immune system. Colostrum can help reverse this by strengthening your immune system, and by putting back actual immune factors that you require to be disease-free. **There's nothing else in the world like colostrum that has the**

**ability to restore DNA and RNA and promote cell growth and tissue repair.**

**Some experts claim it is the ultimate anti-aging food supplement.**
TEN-DAY GREEN SUPERFOOD SMOOTHIE CLEANSE

"Bovine colostrum is safe. Colostrum contains an unprecedented combination of nutritional factors with which to fortify the immune system. It is so harmless, it has been prepared by nature as the first food for infants, intended as their total diet for the first 24 hours."

*"It would be hard to imagine any nutritional substance more natural or beneficial than colostrum. It is safe for internal consumption by children, adults and animals."*
– – Dr. Robert Preston ND, President of the International Institute of nutritional research

Colostrum is not a drug or medicine; it is food. It is a non-toxic, nonallergenic and no side effects super whole food.

Most people feel better right away, but some can go through a healing crisis process. Symptoms can look flu-like, which may include the appearance of fatigue, diarrhea, coughing up phlegm, nausea, skin rash, and even a lowgrade fever. Just hold your course, do not decrease your consumption, in fact, you may want to increase your consumption at this point. This will only happen for a few days. It's your body dumping the toxins that have accumulated for a long time. That were locked in your body's tissues and in the fat deposits that have been suppressing your immune system and encouraging you to be sick and have diseases.

Colostrum is known for being a natural healer and is a safe answer for optimal health today. Many medical research reports presented by doctors and some scientists of major research centers around the world state.

*That the presence of such a wide spectrum of immunoglobulins, antibodies and other immune factors found in colostrum offers tremendous possibilities for the prevention and or recovery from illnesses. Colostrum regulates overactive and underactive immune systems. Colostrum growth factors aid tissue repair by bringing*

*many regenerative anti-aging benefits to us today. They help to
burn fat, increase lean muscle tissue, increase protein synthesis,
build and repair RNA and DNA. They also help with the uptake of
glucose and regenerate nerve, bone, skin and cartilage tissue.*

Colostrum is unprecedented in its ability to fight diseases, improve the quality of life and ameliorate health longitudinally. **It cannot be duplicated in a scientific laboratory.** It's unique combination of growth factors, and immune factors are only possible in this natural whole food product. Colostrum is the first food for all mammals, and nature has designed it perfectly.

*"If it were not for colostrum, the human race wouldn't even exist,"*
~ Dr. Robert Heinerman, Ph.D.

# Chapter 11

## Would You like to Eat All You Can?

### Would You like to Put an End to Yo-Yo Dieting?

That's over, welcome to your new healthy, happy empowering lifestyle!

### New life diet

Would you like to be able to eat all that you want? Of course, you do!

No more up-and-down weight loss programs.

Okay, the ten-day detox diet has passed. If you did all the steps, 7 days of preparation, 10 days of the detox and 4 days for the wind-down, that's 21 days in total. Pat yourself on the back, congratulate yourself, Yahoo! Job well done! It takes approximately 21 days to put a new habit into place. You're there, now move forward and solidify your new dietary habits and lifestyle with the following information. Patients notice certain milestones in feeling better, sense of smell, more weight loss, increased muscle size, increased breast size, increased stamina, mental capacity and many other benefits. I and other patients have noticed a lot of improvement at a three months mark, a six months mark and one year. When you look back, you will be so happy you don't feel the way you used to anymore, and you'll enjoy your new body, mind and attitude.

I was working in the high Andean mountains of South America, in a town called Cusco in the country of Peru. It is a fantastic, beautiful place with more than 5000 years of recorded history of people living there. I loved to eat in the markets, and I noticed that during their corn harvest time, the farmers would come in and eat large amounts of this dish call Toccoo Toccoo. They said it made them strong and kept them going all through the harvest time. Keep in mind that these guys are going out, cutting down the stocks of corn, bailing them up into large bundles and hauling them on their backs. A lot of weight and heavy, hard work. What did they eat you ask? This energy staple food was beans and rice with a few local herbs and spices, and I

49

found it very delicious. I suggested they eat meat before harvest time. I was shocked when they told me that it took away from their ability to work, and they ate that at the celebration party when all was done with lots of beer!

Now that the 10 days are over, do you love your new body? Do you feel great? Do you love where your health is going? Would you like to take it to the next level? Of course you do, let's get going. Here is a list of the proven foods that you're going to want to put in your diet, without starving yourself or eating some crazy unusual foods. Some may be new to you, but others will be old staples. You can still eat pasta and pizza, and some are your favorite dishes, but just make sure you know what flours they're made from.

You may find this surprisingly simple, here are what to include, what not to include and why:

**Animal proteins:** Animal proteins are high on the food chain, Because they are high on the food chain, there's a cumulative buildup of pesticides, modified feedstock, and animal injections that all end up in the meat. Animal proteins trigger cancer. It could be called a dirty diet! Lower on the food chain are quality carbohydrates and vegetables. Hence, they have a little or no chemicals in them when we receive them compared to animal products. These could be called a clean diet.

Additionally, animals are given doses of medications to prevent them from being sick because if animals get sick, we can get the sickness from their products such as meat and eggs. Some examples are the bird flu or the mad cow disease. However, with vegetables, when the plants are sick, we cannot contract the vegetable's sickness. Another reason you want to stick with nonanimal proteins.

This diet is based on quality carbohydrates and starches. Quality carbohydrates come from plants and the sun, and that equals sugar. I know sugar sounds funny. However this type of sugar gives you long lasting energy, unlike the highly processed sugar, were accustomed to eating or the overconsumption of fruit. There's no starch or carbs in animals, so it is not a real source. Also, healthy starches and carbs are very low in fat and are usually between 1 and 8%. They do not contain any human pathogens such as salmonella or E. coli. The plant kingdom is different and doesn't transfer their diseases to humans or the animal kingdom. Quality carbohydrates do not store poisonous chemicals such as DDT or methyl-mercury. Clean carbohydrates are a complete protein, you'll never have to think about eating enough protein, it's just natural.

In 1928, an all potato diet research project was conducted where subjects ate only potatoes and water. The people who volunteered for the experiment not only felt great, but lost weight. And in the end, they did not want to stop eating potatoes.

Studies show people who ate a strict diet of quality carbohydrates and veggies were not overweight 100% of the time!

Let's get you going!

You're going to want to eliminate the following:

Meat

Dairy

No oils except coconut oil

Highly processed foods

Any foods containing artificial sweeteners or corn syrup


The following are items you want to base your diet on:

Most of these are things you can eat your fill of, it is a clean, wholesome food. Once you get accustomed to it, it's very satisfying, but before that, you will most likely go through an adjustment period. How do you create excellent meals? There are thousands of recipes available online.

Eating raw when possible, optimizes the intake of nutritional enzymes. Experts say up to 90% raw is for optimal health. However, do what you can with where you are at.

**Whole grains:**

Millet

Corn

Couscous

Rye

Quinoa

Oats

Barley

Wild and Brown Rice

Buckwheat

Bulgur

Wheat berries

You can also bake with the following unrefined flowers:

Rice

Rye

Soy

Whole wheat

Whole wheat pastry

Potato

Oat

Lima bean

Garbanzo beans

Corn

Buckwheat

Barley

**Quality root carbohydrates:**

Turnips, carrots, and beets are low in calories, and carbohydrates should not be used as staple foods.

Sweet potatoes

Tapioca

Taro root

Water chestnuts

White potatoes

Yams

Sweet potatoes

Celery root

Sunchoke or Jerusalem artichoke

Jicama

Parsnips

Rutabaga roots

Squash:

You want to choose hardy winter squashes because summer squashes are higher in calories and carbohydrate count.

Acorn

Banana

Buttercup

Turban squash

Butternut

Hubbard

Pumpkin

Beans and legumes:

Red kidney

Mung

Pink

Control

White kidney

Idukki

Black

Fava

Chickpeas or garbanzo

Lima

(Soybeans are too high in fat and are used on a regular basis)

Peas and lentils:

Black-eyed

Split yellow

Split and whole green

Brown lentils

Red lentils

Green lentils

**Fruits:**

If you have an issue with triglycerides and cholesterol, please limit your intake of fruit. The average person should have no more than three servings per day, due to the fact it is high in simple sugars.

You can eat almost any organic or clean fruit you like!

## Vegetables:

You can eat almost any organic or clean plant. Eating it raw should be your first choice. Note that sprouted grains are energy packed, and thus a bonus such as lentil, alfalfa, wheat, and mung beans.

## Possible substitutes for the do not eat food list:

Ice cream – frozen juice bars (We make our own) or pure fruit sorbet

Meat – tofu, whole grains, beans and healthy pasta

Milk – water, freshly made fruit juice, almond milk (limited amounts), freshly made vegetable juice, or tea and rice milk

Cheese – nut based and soy cheeses

Vegetable oils for cooking – coconut oil, mashed bananas, applesauce, and water

Vegetable oils for consumption – avocados, nuts and coconut oil

White refined flour – whole-grain flours

Black teas and coffee – cereal beverages, hot water with lemon and noncaffeinated herbal teas

Sodas – water and decaffeinated sun tea

One of our favorites, and a staple around our home

Feel free to change the contents to your liking, there is no limit to the varieties of these recipes. It is very satisfying and gives you long-term energy. You can always decide what to put in and how much.


## Tiida's Thai Beans and Rice

In one bowl serving put in the following

Put in approximately 1 tablespoon of dry shredded seaweed in the bottom of the bowl (many varieties to choose from)

Half or less of brown rice

Half or less of a type of cooked bean. For example, red kidney with some of the broth

Dry cayenne pepper or Asian dried peppers or fresh chili peppers to taste

Fresh ground black pepper we like the telli cherry variety

Half a tablespoon of premium brand fish sauce from Thailand

About 1 tablespoon of premium brand oyster sauce from Thailand

Nuts, one or two of the following cashew nuts, almonds, walnuts, sunflower seeds

Let it sit for a few minutes in the seaweed, and will absorb the liquid broth, and then mix it and enjoy :-)

> *"Processed foods not only extend the shelf life, but they extend the waistline as well."*
>
> ~ Karen Sessions

Now it's time to get started, flip to the next page and find out what your next step is to creating a new you.

# Chapter 12

## Ready, Set Action!

Okay, it's time to get going.

> *New ideas you must take action within 24 hours over 24 hours equals a 50% chance you will do it after that a 2% chance you will do it.*
>
> – – Bill Gates

Start reducing the following items, and by the end of the week, they should be out of your diet. If you think this is too fast for your personal needs, then take two weeks or more. Remember, this is a long-term investment.

Stimulants = coffee, alcohol, and chocolate

Animal protein = beef, chicken, seafood

Valueless carbohydrates = donuts, pastries and other junk foods

Tobacco = chewing tobacco or cigarettes (Wow! This is a significant subject, you understand it is not part of a healthy lifestyle, it's your choice) Things to start right away that will help you out:

Order your colostrum

Order your jumper

Until your little jumper shows up, start exercising every morning and evening. A 15-minute walk is just fine. Note that if you have not been previously following any exercise routine, please just start with two minutes per time and add two minutes on per day. That will make it much easier to be to get going.

You should start the hydrotherapy today! As soon as you finish this book, jump in the shower!

### Summary

Now you understand that you can lose weight, feel better, increase your stamina and even reduce or eliminate medication. You also understand why it's not your fault. Our factory foods have been taunting us with salt, sugar, fat and MSG, so we will just keep eating and eating and eating with the negative nutritional benefit. Now you understand you can turn that around by eliminating these so-called foods groups, or as I call them plastic foods. At this point, you should also understand that if you don't stop the standard American diet, your chances of dying of one of the top 15 diseases in the USA are pretty high. There are only five steps to get you there

**Detox:**

1.     This is a ten-day superfood green smoothie program that will help you eliminate toxic waste and flood your body with the desired nutrients it has been missing.

2.     Adequate intake of water to help flush out the toxins is vital for this transition.

3.     Hot and cold hydrotherapy, this not only helps with the detoxing through the skin, it will also energize and help you sleep like a baby.

4.     Using the rebounder for pumping the lymph nodes and the twist motion which helps detox internal organs.

Exercise: A proper exercise that will help you during the detox and after. You can also use an alternative method that suits your needs.

Meditation: You learned how this would help you de-stress, improve your mental capacities, enhance your behavior and take years off your life.

Superfood: You learned about bovine colostrum whole superfood, its ability to rebuild your body immune system and take you as close as you can get to a fountain of youth potion. And that you will most likely not require any nutritional supplements if you eat healthy clean food.

Green superfood smoothies: This is the fuel that makes this program work, it will help you reset your body clock not to crave junk food, and it is the start of a new all-you-can-eat diet program that will be advantageous to your health.

You have also come to understand that there are 250,000 years of history of fit and trim folks who lived on clean carbs, veggies and fruits, with little or no meat. And also the fact that Asian doctors have been treating patients for more than 2000 years with fasting programs.

Dr. George has set you up for maximum success with the one week before preparation pointers. His assistance with your reduction or elimination of some of the big culprits that have been putting toxins into your body. Your four-day wind down after the cleanse which helps you transition to a new healthy food lifestyle without losing any of the benefits you gained from the detox program.

Anything that you want to do, be or have is possible.

When I was 24 years old, I was out of shape, unhealthy, scatterbrained and had an incurable disease. Now I'm over 55, my blood work, and my physicals show that I'm much younger than the average person of my age. The children in our neighborhood see the doctor at least three or four times a year for different ailments. My three-year-old daughter eats are same foods that we do, and even with a little cheating of some ice cream, or a little sweet by strangers with good intentions, she has never had to go to the doctor! Never!

I would like you to imagine for a moment how your life would be with your ideal weight, body shape, stamina, mental clarity and a great feeling every day. Imagine that? Think how you can be of more benefit to your family, your friends and your community. What type of legacy would you like to leave behind? You can do this, hundreds of thousands have done it before you.

Would you like to help others?

## Paying it forward

*"The first way to pay it forward is by writing a review of this book to let others know about the benefits you got from it. It only takes a few moments. This will not only help others reach their health, happiness and fitness goals. It is incredibly rewarding for me to know how much my work has benefited others, as well as learning any new ways I can improve.... This way, you can help empower others in the way this "ten-day green smoothie cleanse" has empowered you."*

*Leave your review on Amazon at*

TEN-DAY GREEN SUPERFOOD SMOOTHIE CLEANSE: By Marcus D. Norman and Dr. George Della Pietra N.D.

If you would like to contact Dr. George or Marcus D Norman with any success stories or would like to be put on our free book list when they are available, please contact at marcusdnorman@gmail.com

I would recommend that you read this bestseller from Royce Cardiff publishing house during your detox program. Enclosed is a sample chapter. I find it transformational, inspirational and empowering.

## Chapter 1
## Forever Happy Life  Self-Compassion

The reason why this book came about is that I have seen so many people in the world who could be even happier; many of them have great ups and downs and big events, and are very happy for a period of time, and then they crash. I have seen the same outrageous joy in my life, only to be followed later by a deep depression and a lot of self-loathing. Damn, that sucked.

I've had the good fortune of being able to invest a small fortune and thousands of hours studying self-improvement and religion through books, tapes, DVDs, seminar classes, retreats, consulting with gurus, and so on. I have spent time with many experts in many fields of extreme selfimprovement and spiritually centered practices. For example, Time with Hot Coals Walker, Tony Robbins, and Hugging Trees Naked with Native Americans! From Buddhist to Baptists! I went on two different ten-day retreats without speaking, ate vegetarian and meditated for five to six hours per day! I've stayed in a multitude of locations, from sleeping on a cement bed with a wooden pillow to luxury hotels with top self-help gurus at $4000 per weekend. I have not done it all; however, I have done enough.

I have seen that many people do not see the big picture. They seem to know nothing about happiness; they don't understand that they have control over their own being. Many of the teachings around the world can get you to the door of greater happiness. However, it is your job, and only your job, to open that door. If you do the correct things, it need not be difficult. Also, it need not take a long time. I have met a few people who have spent their whole lives seeking the truth. I met a 70-year-old English monk who had spent four hours a day meditating for more than 40 years behind the walls of monasteries. He seemed to me to be one of the most unhappy persons I've ever met; it was very easy to see in his dropping wax like face. I'm going to show you, in this book, how, in a very short time (as quickly as twenty-four hours), you can have much more happiness in your life, and how to keep that happiness.

I retired at the age of 47, healthy, happy, and madly in love! I live in a very beautiful place and have an amazing lifestyle. I am also very successful by most people's standards. What did I learn, and how will it benefit you? I spent countless hours working on myself. Were some of the things I paid a lot of money for worthless, a waste of time, and just plain junk? Yes, many things were and I will save you the heartache of going through that. Did all this educational stuff help me? Yes, of course! Is the information new and revolutionary? The information found in my book is what I have learned from great teachers, sages, poets, ministers, monks, and drunks; my personal observations and life itself. If you have done a lot of personal selfdevelopment, it's possible some of this is not new to you (except maybe for Chapter 7, the ZONE), however, it may be of great benefit to you as a simple reminder of what works and how to get there simpler and quicker. If you're new to self-development, this simple information will change the way you see everything. It's possible to go through many paradigm shifts like peeling the layers of an onion. The good news is many of these of educational programs were fantastic, and I had many paradigm shifts throughout the years. You do not need to spend the next 32 years and your retirement fund to get the results I did. That's why I put this information together; to make it much easier, and to give you the shortest, quickest, most effective way to LongLasting Happiness. It can be yours, in a very, very short time; possibly in the next few days!

If you can do three things, you can get more happiness!

I've simplified and laser-focused them; whittled them down to give you just the meat. Believe it: this information is enough to change your life—quickly.

Some people ask me if I'm perfect, do I do all the things I suggest in my books? Very funny. No way; I'm a human just like you. I have my moments, just figuring things out. However, I've had many successes on this incredible journey and I have been blessed with time, money, and the willingness to experience and experiment the different aspects of this amazing life on Planet Earth!

I give you a lot of kudos for investing in yourself and reading this book. It shows that you are above average, and have the desire and drive to want more true happiness from this amazing life.

Congratulations!

> *"Some of my greatest teachers were ministers, monks, and drunks."*
> — Jimmy Jerome Johnson

Order your copy today
HAPPINESS LIFE: Your Simple Proven 3 Step Guide to Making Radical SelfImprovement Today!

> *"Be you and change the world"*
> — Gary M. Douglas

> *This is your last chance. After this, there is no turning back. You take the blue pill - the story ends, you wake up in your bed and believe whatever you want to believe. You take the red pill - you stay in Wonderland and I show you how deep the rabbit-hole goes*
> --Morpheus from the movie Matrix

## Highly recommend read list

Eat. Nourish. Glow.: 10 easy steps for losing weight, looking younger & feeling healthier by Amelia Freer

10-Day Green Smoothie Cleanse: Lose Up to 15 Pounds in 10 Days! by JJ Smith

NOTE: You will see that I do not agree with all of her ideas, however it is very inspirational reading it to help you on your journey.

Superfood Smoothies: 100 Delicious, Energizing & Nutrient-dense Recipes by Julie Morris

A well done hardcover that will be a welcome addition to your creative kitchen. It is a must have.

The Blood Sugar Solution 10-Day Detox Diet: Activate Your Body's Natural Ability to Burn Fat and Lose Weight Fast by Mark Hyman

Supply List

Jumper

As you establish a consistent rebound exercise program, you will receive benefits that far exceed the cost of the unit. When ordering, I recommend the unit with the bar included. Rebounderjoy.com

For a $40 worth of bonus gifts.

BodyBoost bovine colostrum powder is available for a 50% discount at Amazon.com

All other products in this book should be available on Amazon, or your local health food store or supermarket. Try to use organic produce where possible, give it a thorough washing before consuming.

# 101 Smoothie Recipes

I'm going to re-include the basic smoothie template from chapter 4. This is not rocket science. After a few weeks, you'll be an expert and be teaching your friends.

As stated earlier, there's thousands of ways to make a smoothie and many ingredients are available. Use your judgment and experiment. The 101 smoothie recipes below are not intended to be used during the detox cleanse diet. Use them as a frame of reference, for you to explore the unlimited possibilities.

Enjoy!

**Smoothie template to create five smoothies per day and at one time.**
2 cups of water (adjust amount as needed to help it liquefy)
Oil = can be 1 tablespoon of coconut oil, fish oil or nuts and seeds, walnuts, almonds, cashews, sesame seeds, etc.
25% fruit = apples and berries, etc.
75% green leafy vegetables = spinach, kale, mixed baby greens, etc.
4 tablespoons of 100% whole bovine colostrum powder (after the cleanse just 1tablespoon per 16oz smoothie)
2 tablespoons of vegetable protein, hemp, pea powder (protein = no hunger) (not necessary after fast)

Typically, you want to pick just one from each following categories below. Here are some basic rules:

1. As much as possible, always use fresh ingredients, they could also be frozen. However, NO canned, bottled or preserved foods.
2. No dairy
3. No dairy like substances, like almond or soy milk (Highly processed and have sugar)
4. Very little to no sweeteners
5. About 1cups of fruits to 4 cups of packed greens and 1 cup of water

**Liquid base:**
1 cup of water
1 cup of green tea

1 cup of your favorite healthy tea

## Healthy oils:

Pick one per recipe. Organic, nuts must be raw and oils must be cold pressed

2 tablespoons of coconut oil 2
  tablespoons of flaxseed oil
  Quarter cup of raw cashews
One and half avocado
2 tablespoons of flaxseed (sprouted is even much better)
2 tablespoons of Chia seed (sprouted is even much better)

## Fruits:

It is best to keep fruits below 25% of the ingredients. Feel free to vary the amount according to the recipe. The amount listed below are just suggestions.

One Apple with skin
Half of a banana
One-quarter of a peeled orange
One-quarter of a lime
One-quarter of a lemon
One-quarter of a pineapple
Grapefruit
Blueberries
Pomegranates
Raspberries
Pears with the skin
Oranges
Kiwi
Cantaloupe
Apricots

## Veggies:

Brussels sprouts
Cauliflower
Book joy
Beets
Pumpkin
Kale
Broccoli
Celery
Cucumber with the skin

All leafy greens, for example, arugula, spinach, and baby Kale  Collard greens

Spring greens

Swiss chard

Green cabbage

Arugula

Barley grass

Sprouts

Dandelion greens

Mustard greens

Mint (use in smaller quantities)

Parsley (use in smaller quantities)

Cilantro (coriander)

Mixed baby leaf salad mix

Carrots (small amounts)

Tomatoes

## Super foods:

Always put in 1 teaspoon colostrum per 16oz smoothie and one of the following.

Kale

¼ teaspoon Camu Camu

Maca

Wheat grass

Avocado

Hemp protein powder

2 tablespoons raw cocoa powder or nibs

2 tablespoons Chia seeds

2 tablespoons coconut oil

1/8 teaspoon to half a teaspoon of cayenne pepper (adjust to tolerance level of heat)

Goji beans

## Nuts:

5 to 10 raw almonds (soak overnight)

5 to 10 raw walnuts (soak overnight) 5 to 10 raw cashew nuts (soaked overnight) Protein powders:

Pea protein powder

Hemp powder

Rice powder

**Sweeteners:**

Stevia

**Other Ingredients:**

Mesquite Powder

Cayenne pepper dry

Medical mushrooms


This is your basic detox smoothie cleanse template. After the cleanse, you can vary the amounts of the ingredients, for example, add more fruit at subtraction and substitute ingredients.

There are thousands upon thousands of smoothie recipes. You can create all kinds of recipes. There's a beautiful hardback book available from Amazon see my resource section. Some for losing weight, healing, helping with cold and sickness symptoms, giving you more energy or simply making a wonderful dessert!

Enjoy

## Rose Mary's Chamomile, Peach, Spinach and Ginger Smoothie

**Ingredients**

2 packed handfuls of fresh spinach

2 peaches, skinned, stone removed

2 teaspoons of fresh ginger

2 teaspoons of colostrum

2 teaspoons of wheat germ (optional)

2 chamomile tea bags

2 tablespoons of flaxseed

¼ teaspoon of camu camu

10 raw almonds (soaked overnight)

Place the teabags in a cup, cover with one and half cup (350ml) of boiling water.

Allow to cool, Remove bag and place tea in blender with all remaining ingredients and blend until smooth. This should make about two 12 oz. (350ml) servings.

Enjoy!

## Sparkling Frozen Blueberry Smoothie

Ingredients

150g (1 cup) frozen blueberries

2 cups of mustard greens

4 tablespoons of coconut oil

2 tablespoons of honey (optional)

2 teaspoons of colostrum

2 tablespoons of wheat germ

4 tablespoons of whey protein powder

10 raw almonds (soaked overnight)

Place all ingredients in a blender and blend until smooth.

This should make about two 12 oz. (350ml) servings.

Enjoy!

If you prefer not to eat a proper meal before sport, this smoothie is the ideal solution, especially if you get pre-event jitters. You can also use frozen strawberries, raspberries or mango.

## Macie's High-fiber Cleansing Smoothie

**Ingredients**

500g (2 cups) of papaya, peeled and roughly chopped

2 small cucumbers, roughly chopped

2 handfuls of spinach

½ cup of plain coconut water or water

2 teaspoons of colostrum

2 oranges, peeled

Quarter a cup of raw cashews (soaked overnight)

Place all ingredients in a blender and blend until smooth.

This should make about two 12 oz. (350ml) servings.

Enjoy!

## Suzanne's Mixed Berry with Broccoli Smoothie

**Ingredients**

150g (2/3 cup) of strawberries, hulled, and roughly chopped

½ (75 grams) cup of fresh or frozen raspberries

1 cup of fresh broccoli

1 cup of spring green lettuce

1 cup (200ml) of mint tea

2 teaspoons of colostrum

1 tablespoon of maple syrup (optional)

4 ice cubes

¼ teaspoon of Camu Camu

10 raw walnuts( soak overnight)

2 tablespoons of sunflower oil

Place all ingredients in a blender and blend until smooth.

This should make about two 12 oz. (350ml) servings.

Enjoy!

## Refreshing Peach & Cucumber Mint Smoothie

**Ingredients**

½ cup of fresh peach (diced)
½ cup of fresh cucumber
2 handfuls of spinach
2 apples
½ cup of green tea
2 teaspoons of colostrum
2 tablespoons of fresh mint leaves
5 to 10 raw walnuts (soaked overnight)
2 tablespoons of flaxseed
1 cup of ice cubes( about 200 ml)

Place all ingredients in a blender and blend until smooth.

This should make about two 12 oz. (350ml) servings.

Enjoy!

## Barbara's Carrot Smoothie

1 cup of coconut water or cool water
4 ice cubes
1 lemon
4 carrots cubed
1 orange, peeled
1 tablespoon of flaxseed
½ teaspoon of cayenne pepper
2 teaspoons of colostrum
2 tablespoons of coconut oil
10 raw walnuts (soaked overnight)

Place all ingredients in a blender and blend until smooth.

This should make about two 12 oz. (350ml) servings.

Enjoy!

## Green Monster Smoothie

### Ingredients
1 ½ cup of coconut water or water (350ml)
1 cup of spring greens
1 banana
2 cups of fresh spinach
1 cup of ice cubes

2 teaspoons of colostrum

2 tablespoons of chia seed

10 raw walnuts (soaked overnight)

Place all ingredients in a blender and blend until smooth.

This should make about two 12 oz. (350ml) servings.

Enjoy!

## Martha's Spinach and Kale Smoothie

### Ingredients

2 packed hand full of fresh spinach

1 ½ cup of water

2 tablespoons of chia seeds

2 kale leaves

1 peeled banana

2 teaspoons of colostrum

¼ teaspoon of camu camu

2 tablespoons of coconut oil

10 cashew nuts (soaked overnight)

Place all ingredients in a blender and blend until smooth.

This should make about two 12 oz. (350ml) servings.

Enjoy!

## Barbara's Carrot with Collard Greens Smoothie

1 large carrot, peeled and diced

1 packed handful of collard greens (stem removed)

1 ½ cups of green tea

½ banana, peeled

2 teaspoons of colostrum

1 teaspoon ground allspice

¼ teaspoon Of cayenne pepper

10 raw almonds (soaked overnight)

2 tablespoons of coconut oil

Place all ingredients in a blender and blend until smooth.

This should make about two 12 oz. (350ml) servings.

Enjoy!

## Cool Green Smoothie

1 ½ cups of cold water
1 packed hand full of baby kale
8 fresh mint leaves
½ mango, peeled and pitted
1 lemon, peeled
2 teaspoons of coconut oil
2 teaspoons of colostrum
¼ teaspoon of camu camu
10 raw walnuts (soaked overnight)

Place all ingredients in a blender and blend until smooth.

This should make about two 12 Oz. (350ml) servings.

Enjoy!

## Slimy Pumpkin Smoothie

2 cups (about 16 Oz ) of diced pumpkin
1 ½ cups ( 12 Oz  ) of coconut water or water
1 cup of diced papaya
2 teaspoons of ground cinnamon
¼ cup of maple syrup (optional)
2 teaspoons of colostrum
2 tablespoons of wheat germ
2 tablespoons of flaxseed
10 raw almonds (soaked overnight)

Place all ingredients in a blender and blend until smooth.

This should make about two 12 oz. (350ml) servings.

Enjoy!

## Lean Green Smoothie

Ingredients
1 ½ cups of cubed honeydew melon
1 ½ cups of ice cubes (12 Oz)
½ cup of green grapes

1 cucumber

½ cup of broccoli florets

1 sprig of fresh mint

2 tablespoons of coconut oil

2 teaspoons of colostrum

¼ teaspoons of camu camu

10 raw cashew nuts (soaked overnight)

Place all ingredients in a blender and blend until smooth.

This should make about two 12 oz. (350ml) servings.

Enjoy!

## Don't knock it until you try the Zucchini spinach and Banana with Nut smoothie

1  zucchini

2  large ripe bananas, peeled

2 handfuls of fresh spinach

1 ½ cups (350ml) of green tea

2 tablespoons of cocoa powder

¼ cup of chopped peanuts

1 medium packet of stevia (optional)

10 raw almonds (soaked overnight)

2 teaspoons of colostrum

2 tablespoons of coconut oil

¼ teaspoon of camu camu

Place all ingredients in a blender and blend until smooth.

This should make about two 12 oz. (350ml) servings.

Enjoy!

## Mouthwatering Strawberry Mustard Green Smoothie

2 packed handfuls of mustard greens

½ cup of green tea

1 cup of coconut water or water

4 ice cubes

6 strawberries

½ banana, cut into chunks

10 raw almonds (soaked overnight)

¼ maple syrup (optional)

2 teaspoons of colostrum

¼ teaspoon of cayenne pepper

2 tablespoons of coconut oil

Place all ingredients in a blender and blend until smooth.

This should make about two 12 Oz. (350ml) servings.

Enjoy!

## Janie's Amazing Zucchini Smoothie

Ingredients

2 zucchinis

5 ice cubes

1 orange (peeled)

2 tablespoons of maple syrup (optional)

1 cup of coconut water or cool water

2 teaspoons of coconut oil

2 teaspoons of colostrum

2 teaspoons of Maca

10 raw walnuts (soaked overnight)

¾ teaspoon of vanilla extract

Place all ingredients in a blender and blend until smooth.

This should make about two 12 oz. (350ml) servings.

Enjoy!

## Jane's Kale Orange Banana Smoothie

Ingredients

3 kale leaves

1 orange, peeled

½ cup of water

1 cup of green tea

1 ripe banana, peeled

10 raw walnuts (soaked overnight)

2 teaspoons of colostrum

2 teaspoons of chia seeds

2 tablespoons of coconut oil

Place all ingredients in a blender and blend until smooth.

This should make about two 12 oz. (350ml) servings.

Enjoy!

## Cinnamon Spinach healthy smoothie

1 apple
2 packed handfuls of fresh spinach
1 teaspoon of ground cinnamon
½ cup of ice
1 cup of herbal tea
2 teaspoons of colostrum
Wheatgrass (use according to preference)
2 tablespoons of coconut oil
10 raw cashew nuts (soaked overnight)

Place all ingredients in a blender and blend until smooth.

This should make about two 12 oz. (350ml) servings.

Enjoy!

## 'Yam Yam!' Smoothie

2 medium yams
2 packed handfuls of fresh arugula
1 cup of green tea
2 teaspoons of colostrum
¼ teaspoons of camu camu
10 raw walnuts (soaked overnight)
2 cups of ice cubes
1 teaspoon of honey ( optional)
1 ripe banana, peeled
2 tablespoons of mesquite powder
2 teaspoons of coconut oil

Place all ingredients in a blender and blend until smooth.

This should make about two 12 oz. (350ml) servings.

Enjoy!

## Janie's Amazing Smoothie

2 zucchinis, cubed

5 ice cubes

1 handful of spinach

1 cup of coconut water or cool water

1 orange

2 tablespoons of stevia

¾ teaspoon of vanilla extract

¼ teaspoon of camu camu

2 teaspoons of colostrum

10 raw almonds (soaked overnight)

2 tablespoons of coconut oil

2 teaspoons of chia seeds

Place all ingredients in a blender and blend until smooth.

This should make about two 12 oz. (350ml) servings.

Enjoy!

## Aunt Marie's Cucumber and Kale with Ginger Smoothie

1 cup of roughly chopped cucumber

1 handful of baby kale

1 apple

1 cup of water

½ cup of ice cubes

2 teaspoons of colostrum

1 tablespoon of fresh ginger

2 tablespoons of coconut oil

¼ teaspoons of camu camu

10 raw walnuts (soaked overnight)

Place all ingredients in a blender and blend until smooth.

This should make about two 12 oz. (350ml) servings.

Enjoy!

## Lucy's Cabbage & Apple with Green Tea Smoothie

1/1 handful of fresh spinach

½ cabbage, cubed

½ apple

1 cup of green tea

6 ice cubes

1 teaspoon of flaxseed
½ lemon, peeled
2 teaspoons of colostrum
1 tablespoon of cayenne pepper
10 raw almonds (soaked overnight)
2 tablespoons of coconut oil

Place all ingredients in a blender and blend until smooth.

This should make about two 12 oz. (350ml) servings.

Enjoy!

## Tantalizing Sweet Potato and Banana with Kale Smoothie

1 large sweet potato
1 banana, peeled
2 packed handfuls of kale
1 ½ cups (350ml) of herbal tea
10 raw cashew nuts (soaked overnight)
2 teaspoons of colostrum
2 teaspoons of Maca
2 tablespoons of coconut oil
¼ teaspoon of ground cinnamon

Place all ingredients in a blender and blend until smooth.

This should make about two 12 oz. (350ml) servings.

Enjoy!

## Hala Kahiki Green Smoothie

1 cup of herbal tea
2 packed handful of fresh spinach
1 packed handful of kale
1 cup of red seedless grapes
1 cup of ice
2 tablespoons of coconut oil
2 teaspoons of colostrum 2 tablespoons of
flaxseed
10 raw cashew nuts (soaked overnight)
½ teaspoons of cayenne pepper (reduce if necessary) Place all ingredients in a
blender and blend until smooth.

This should make about two 12 oz. (350ml) servings.

Enjoy!

## Jumping Ginger Smoothie

1 ½ (350 ml) cups of cold water
1 avocado, peeled and pitted
½ cup of fresh parsley
1 apple
2 carrots, cut into chunks
1 lemon, peeled
1 packed handful of kale
1 (1 inch) piece fresh ginger root, or more to taste
2 ice cubes
2 teaspoons of flaxseed
2 tablespoons of coconut oil
2 teaspoons of colostrum
10 raw almonds (soaked overnight)

Place all ingredients in a blender and blend until smooth.

This should make about two 12 oz. (350ml) servings.

Enjoy!

## Refreshing Green Tea with Blueberry and Dandelion Greens Smoothie

1 ½ handful of dandelion greens
¾ cup of green tea
8 ice cubes
¼ banana, peeled
½ cup of frozen blueberries
2 tablespoons of coconut oil
2 teaspoons of colostrum
¼ teaspoon of cayenne pepper
10 raw cashew nuts (soaked overnight)

Place all ingredients in a blender and blend until smooth.

This should make about two 12 Oz. (350ml) servings.

Enjoy!

## Spinach with Ginger and Cucumber Healthy Smoothie

1 cucumber, diced
¼ mango, peeled
2 packed handfuls of fresh spinach
½ cup of chamomile tea
1 cup of cool water
1 tablespoon of ground cinnamon
2 teaspoons of colostrum
¼ teaspoon of camu camu
2 teaspoons of ground ginger
10 raw almonds (soaked overnight)
2 tablespoons of coconut oil

Place all ingredients in a blender and blend until smooth.

This should make about two 12 oz. (350ml) servings.

Enjoy!

## Cucumber-Honeydew Smoothie

1 cucumber
2 cups of cubed honeydew melon
1 orange, peeled
8 sprigs of fresh mint (or amount to taste)
10 raw walnuts (soaked overnight)
2 tablespoons of coconut oil
2 teaspoons of chia seeds
6 ice cubes
2 teaspoons of colostrum
1 cup of water

Place all ingredients in a blender and blend until smooth.

This should make about two 12 oz. (350ml) servings.

Enjoy!

## Caribbean Health drink

1 cup of water
1 cup of cubed carrot

2 packed handful of fresh spinach

10 raw almonds (soaked overnight)

1 kiwi, peeled

½ cup of chopped pineapple

2 tablespoons of coconut oil

2 teaspoons of colostrum

¼ teaspoon of camu camu

1 cup of ice cubes

Place all ingredients in a blender and blend until smooth.

This should make about two 12 oz. (350ml) servings.

Enjoy!

## Heavenly Spinach with Fruit Smoothie

2 packed handfuls of baby spinach

½ apple

½ bananas, peeled

1 cup of cubed carrots

½ cup of fresh strawberries

1 cup of herbal tea

5 ice cubes

10 raw cashew nuts (soaked overnight)

2 teaspoons of colostrum

2 tablespoons of cocoa powder

2 tablespoons of coconut oil

Place all ingredients in a blender and blend until smooth.

This should make about two 12 oz. (350ml) servings.

Enjoy!

## Pumpkin Pie Smoothie

1 ½ cups of cubed pumpkin

1 apple

1 ½ cups (350ml) of your favorite tea

1/8 teaspoon of ground nutmeg

10 raw almonds (soaked overnight)

2 teaspoons of colostrum

1 teaspoon of ground cinnamon

2 tablespoons of coconut oil

Wheat grass (use appropriately)

Place all ingredients in a blender and blend until smooth.

This should make about two 12 oz. (350ml) servings.

Enjoy!

## Green Power Mojito Smoothie

1 cup of ice cubes, or as desired

2 packed handfuls of  baby spinach

1 (250ml) cup of water

1 cucumber

1 orange, peeled

10 fresh mint leaves, or more to taste

1 lemon, peeled

1 lime, peeled

10 raw walnuts (soaked overnight)

2 teaspoons of colostrum

¼ teaspoon of camu camu

2 tablespoons of sunflower oil

Place all ingredients in a blender and blend until smooth.

This should make about two 12 oz. (350ml) servings.

Enjoy!

## Green Fruity Smoothie

2 packed handfuls of baby spinach

1 apple

½  bananas, peeled

1 cup of cubed carrot

1 orange, peeled

½  cup of fresh strawberries

1 cup of ice ( about 5 cubes)

2 teaspoons of colostrum

½ teaspoon of cayenne pepper

2 teaspoons of coconut oil

10 raw almonds (soaked overnight)

Place all ingredients in a blender and blend until smooth.

This should make about two 12 oz. (350ml) servings.

Enjoy!

## Thin Mint Green Monster

½ cup of coconut water or cool water
1 cup of herbal tea
2 packed handfuls of fresh spinach
10 leaves fresh mint
¼ cup of raw cacao seeds
10 cashew nuts (soaked overnight)
1 (1 gram) packet of stevia powder (optional)
1 banana, peeled
2 teaspoons of colostrum
¼ teaspoon of camu camu
2 tablespoons of coconut oil
Water, or as needed

Place all ingredients in a blender and blend until smooth.

This should make about two 12 oz. (350ml) servings.

Enjoy!

## Spinach under Mango Cloak Smoothie

1 cup of frozen mango chunks
1 handful of kale
1 ½ cups of cool water
2 handfuls of fresh spinach
½ orange, peeled
10 raw almonds (soaked overnight)
2 tablespoons of coconut oil
2 teaspoons of colostrum
2 tablespoons of chia seeds
1 cup of ice (optional)

Place all ingredients in a blender and blend until smooth.

This should make about two 12 oz. (350ml) servings.

Enjoy!

## Tropical Smoothie with Kale and Broccoli

1 cup of frozen pineapple chunks
1 handful of kale
1 cup of toughly cubed broccoli
1 cup of coconut water
½ cup of cool water
10 raw almonds ( soaked overnight)
2 tablespoons of coconut oil
1 teaspoon of cocoa powder
2 tablespoons of chia seeds

Place all ingredients in a blender and blend until smooth.

This should make about two 12 oz. (350ml) servings.

Enjoy!

## Spicy Pumpkin Protein Smoothie

½ banana, peeled
1 (12oz) cup of pumpkin chunks
2 dates, pitted
1 scoop of vanilla protein powder
½ teaspoon of vanilla extract 2 tablespoons of
coconut oil
1 pinch of ground nutmeg
1 pinch of ground cinnamon
1 pinch of ground cloves
1 pinch of ground ginger
2 teaspoons of colostrum
10 raw walnuts (soaked overnight)

Place all ingredients in a blender and blend until smooth.

This should make about two 12 oz. (350ml) servings.

Enjoy!

## Rosie's Kale, Cucumber with Banana Smoothie

2 handfuls of fresh kale

1 cup of chopped fresh pineapple

½ cucumber chopped

½ banana

2 teaspoons of colostrum

2 teaspoons of chia seeds

¼ cup of frozen blackberries (or more to taste)

2 tablespoons of coconut oil

10 raw walnuts (soaked overnight)

1 cup of mint tea

4 ice cubes

Place all ingredients in a blender and blend until smooth.

This should make about two 12 oz. (350ml) servings.

Enjoy!

## Kiwi Sensation

1 kiwi, peeled

½ cup of kale

¼ mango - peeled, seeded

¼ cup of water

2 handfuls of fresh spinach

2 cups of ice cubes, or as needed

1 cup of tea or water

10 raw almonds (soaked overnight)

2 teaspoons of colostrum

¼ teaspoon of camu camu

2 tablespoons of olive oil

Place all ingredients in a blender and blend until smooth.

This should make about two 12 oz. (350ml) servings.

Enjoy!

## Any Way You Want It Kale Smoothie

2 cups of chopped kale

¼ cup of parsley

1 cup of herbal tea

6 ice cubes

3 tablespoons of peanuts (optional)

½ frozen banana

3 frozen strawberries, or more to taste

1 tablespoon of maple syrup (optional)

2 tablespoons of coconut oil

2 teaspoons of colostrum

2 tablespoons of hemp protein powder

1o raw walnuts (soaked overnight)

Place all ingredients in a blender and blend until smooth.

This should make about two 12 oz. (350ml) servings.

Enjoy!

## Cabbage, Peach, and Carrot Smoothie

¼ cup of grapes

1 cup of sliced frozen peaches

1 cup of chopped cabbage

1 large carrot cubed

10 raw cashew nuts (soaked overnight)

1 cup of ice cubes

1 cup of water or tea(as desired)

2 teaspoons of colostrum

¼ teaspoon of camu camu

2 tablespoons of olive oil

2 tablespoons of maple syrup(optional)

Place all ingredients in a blender and blend until smooth.

This should make about two 12 oz. (350ml) servings.

Enjoy!

## Rosy Rhubarb Smoothie

1 ½ cups of frozen chopped rhubarb

1 small banana

1 handful of fresh kale

½ cup of tea

1 cup of coconut water or water
10 raw almonds (soaked overnight)
3 drops of red food coloring (optional)
2 tablespoons of coconut oil
2 teaspoons of colostrum
2 tablespoons of chia seeds

Place all ingredients in a blender and blend until smooth.

This should make about two 12 oz. (350ml) servings.

Enjoy!

## Banana Pineapple Green Blend

1 cup of chamomile tea
1 ½  packed handfuls of baby spinach leaves
½ cup of water
½ banana
½ cup of chopped frozen pineapple
10 raw almonds (soaked overnight)
2 teaspoons of colostrum
2 tablespoons of coconut oil
¼ teaspoon of cayenne pepper

Place all ingredients in a blender and blend until smooth.

This should make about two 12 oz. (350ml) servings.

Enjoy!

## Aunt Macie's Spinach and Berry Smoothie

1 cup of fresh strawberries
1  orange (peeled)
1 handful of kale
2 packed handful of fresh baby spinach
1 cup of ice
1 cup of tea
10 raw walnuts (soaked overnight)
2 teaspoons of colostrum
¼ teaspoon of camu camu

2 tablespoons of coconut oil

Place all ingredients in a blender and blend until smooth.

This should make about two 12 oz. (350ml) servings.

Enjoy!

## Broccolious smoothie

2 cups of chopped broccoli
1 handful of fresh spinach
1 cup of seedless green grapes, or more to taste
1 small cucumber, cubed
½ cup of water, or as needed
1 cup of chamomile tea
1 lime
2 teaspoons of colostrum
2 tablespoons of olive oil
2 tablespoons of chia seeds
10 raw cashew nuts (soaked overnight)

Place all ingredients in a blender and blend until smooth.

This should make about two 12 oz. (350ml) servings.

Enjoy!

## Quick Kale and Banana Smoothie

2 cups of chopped kale
1 banana
1 cup of herbal tea
5 ice cubes
2 teaspoons of coconut oil
10 raw walnuts (soaked overnight)
Wheat grass
2 teaspoons of colostrum
½ cup of coconut water
½ cup of frozen strawberries

Place all ingredients in a blender and blend until smooth.

This should make about two 12 oz. (350ml) servings.

Enjoy!

## Spicy Pumpkin smoothie

4 ice cubes

1 cup of green tea

1 cup of pumpkin, cubed

1/3 cup of coconut water (optional)

½ banana

1 pinch of ground cinnamon

1 pinch of ground ginger

1 pinch of ground nutmeg

1 pinch of ground allspice

2 teaspoons of colostrum

1 teaspoon of vanilla extract

¼ teaspoon of camu camu

10 raw walnuts (soaked overnight)

2 tablespoons of coconut oil

Place all ingredients in a blender and blend until smooth.

This should make about two 12 oz. (350ml) servings.

Enjoy!

## Mesmerizing Zucchini with Swiss chard Smoothie

1 zucchini, chopped

3 large Swiss chard leaves

1 cup of chilled tea

½ cup of cool water

6 blueberries, or more to taste

2 tablespoons of honey(optional)

1 tablespoon of flaxseeds 2 teaspoons of
colostrum

1 teaspoon of Maca

2 teaspoons of coconut oil

10 raw almonds (soaked overnight)

Place all ingredients in a blender and blend until smooth.

This should make about two 12 Oz. (350ml) servings.

Enjoy!

## Very Orange Smoothie without Oranges

1 mango - peeled, seeded 2 carrots, cut into
chunks
1 yellow bell pepper, chopped
½ red bell pepper, chopped
1 cup of chilled mineral water
½ cup of tea
1 lemon
2 tablespoons of coconut oil
1 teaspoon of honey (optional)
2 teaspoons of colostrum
10 raw walnuts (soaked overnight)
2 teaspoons of chia seeds

Place all ingredients in a blender and blend until smooth.

This should make about two 12 oz. (350ml) servings.

Enjoy!

## Good-To-Go Morning Smoothie

2 packed handfuls of fresh spinach
1 cup of oatmeal
1 ½ cups of green tea
1 apple
2 ice cubes
10 raw cashew nuts (soaked overnight)
2 teaspoons of colostrum
2 tablespoons of coconut oil
¼ teaspoon of camu camu
2 teaspoons of chia seeds

Place all ingredients in a blender and blend until smooth.

This should make about two 12 oz. (350ml) servings.

Enjoy!

## Cool Kale Smoothie

1 cup of green grapes  2 cups of kale
1 cup of spring greens

10 raw almonds (soaked overnight)

1 cup of ice cubes

2 tablespoons of coconut oil

2 teaspoons of colostrum

2 teaspoons of maca

Place all ingredients in a blender and blend until smooth.

This should make about two 12 oz. (350ml) servings.

Enjoy!

## Cabbage with Parsley and Carrot Smoothie

1 cup of roughly chopped cabbage

1 orange, peeled

½ handful of parsley

1 large carrot, peeled and chopped

1 tablespoon of fresh ginger

10 raw cashew nuts (soaked overnight)

1 cup of water

½ cup of ice cubes

2 teaspoons of chia seeds

2 teaspoons of colostrum

2 tablespoons of coconut oil

Place all ingredients in a blender and blend until smooth.

This should make about two 12 oz. (350ml) servings.

Enjoy!

## Pumpkin Apple Pie Smoothie

1 apple

1 cup of water

2/3 cup of herbal tea

2 tablespoons of olive oil  1 cup of
    pumpkin, cubed

1 ½ teaspoons of maple syrup(optional)

¼ teaspoon cayenne pepper

10 raw walnuts (soaked overnight)

2 teaspoons of colostrum

2/3 cup of ice cubes

2 teaspoons of chia seeds

Place all ingredients in a blender and blend until smooth.

This should make about two 12 oz. (350ml) servings.

Enjoy!

## Aunt Martha's Pumpkin with Cucumber Smoothie

1 banana, peeled
3 whole frozen strawberries
1 ½ cucumbers
1 cup of herbal tea
½ teaspoon of cayenne pepper
2 teaspoons of colostrum
½ cup of pumpkin cubes
1 stevia packet (optional)
2 teaspoons of coconut oil
¼ teaspoon of ground cinnamon
10 raw almonds (soaked overnight)
1 pinch of ground nutmeg
¼ teaspoon of camu camu
4 ice cubes

Place all ingredients in a blender and blend until smooth. This should make about two 12 oz. (350ml) servings. Enjoy!

## Easy Pumpkin Pie Smoothie

1 cup of pumpkin cubes

1 cup of green tea

4 ice cubes

1 banana

1 cinnamon graham cracker

2 teaspoons of wheat germ

2 tablespoons of coconut oil 1

teaspoon of vanilla extract

2 teaspoons of colostrum

1 teaspoon of pumpkin pie spice

½ teaspoon of ground cinnamon

10 raw walnuts (soaked overnight)

Place all ingredients in a blender and blend until smooth. This should make about two 12 oz. (350ml) servings.

1 pinch of

ground cinnamon

Enjoy!

## The Orange Power Smoothie

1 cup of coconut water or cool water

4 ice cubes

1 lemon

4 carrots cubed

1 orange, peeled

1 tablespoon of flaxseed

2 teaspoons of chia seeds

2 teaspoons of colostrum

2 tablespoons of coconut oil

1 pinch of salt

10 raw almonds (soaked overnight)

4 pitted dates

Place all ingredients in a blender and blend until smooth.

This should make about two 12 oz. (350ml) servings.

Enjoy!

## Endless Energy smoothie

1 cup of green tea
5 cubes of ice
1 handful of baby kale
1 packed handful of fresh spinach
1 kiwi, peeled and chopped
½ cup of chopped pineapple
2 teaspoons of colostrum
2 tablespoons of coconut oil
2 teaspoons of pea protein powder
2 teaspoons of chia seeds
10 raw cashew nuts (soaked overnight)

Place all ingredients in a blender and blend until smooth.

This should make about two 12 oz. (350ml) servings.

Enjoy!

## Carrot Cake Smoothie

1 large carrot, peeled and diced
¼ mango, peeled
1 cucumber, chopped
½ cup of vanilla tea
1 cup of cool water
1 tablespoon of ground cinnamon
2 teaspoons of colostrum
1 teaspoon of ground allspice
¼ teaspoon of camu camu
1 teaspoon of ground ginger
10 raw almonds (soaked overnight)
2 tablespoons of olive oil

Place all ingredients in a blender and blend until smooth.

This should make about two 12 oz. (350ml) servings.

Enjoy!

## Eye-catching Beet and Berry Smoothie

1 packed handful of fresh spinach
1 beet, peeled and cut into quarters
½ cucumber, cubed

½ cup of dandelion greens

½ cup of frozen unsweetened red raspberries

½ cup of frozen blueberries

½ tablespoons of cayenne pepper

10 raw almonds (soaked overnight)

½ cup of ice cubes

1 ½ cups of tea

2 teaspoons of colostrum

2 tablespoons of coconut oil

Place all ingredients in a blender and blend until smooth.

This should make about two 12 oz. (350ml) servings.

Enjoy!

## Healthy Caesar Smoothie

2 large tomatoes

2 handfuls of loosely packed fresh spinach

1 lemon

1 banana, peeled

1 pinch of ground black pepper

2 teaspoons of colostrum

2 teaspoons of chia seeds

1 cup of water

4 ice cubes

10 raw walnuts (soaked overnight)

2 tablespoons of coconut oil

Place all ingredients in a blender and blend until smooth.

This should make about two 12 oz. (350ml) servings.

Enjoy!

## Stellar Kale Smoothie

2 handfuls of fresh kale

1 cup of chopped fresh pineapple

8 pitted dates

1 tablespoon of vanilla extract

2 teaspoons of colostrum

2 teaspoons of chia seeds

¼ cup of frozen blackberries (to taste)

2 tablespoons of coconut oil

10 raw cashew nuts (soaked overnight)

1 cup of mint tea

4 ice cubes

Place all ingredients in a blender and blend until smooth.

This should make about two 12 oz. (350ml) servings.

Enjoy!

## Veggie, Fruit, and Nut Nutritious Green Smoothie

1 ½ cups of baby spinach leaves

1 cup of shredded carrots

½ cup of sliced raw beet

½ pear, cored and chopped

½ banana

1 cup of coconut water or water

½ cup of green tea

¼ cup of walnut halves

¼ cup of whole almonds

2 tablespoons of coconut oil

1 tablespoon of honey (optional)

2 teaspoons of colostrum

½ teaspoon of ground cinnamon

¼ teaspoon of camu camu

Place all ingredients in a blender and blend until smooth.

This should make about two 12 oz. (350ml) servings.

Enjoy!

## Winter Refresher Green Smoothie

1 cup of water

½ cup of green tea

2 loosely packed handfuls of fresh spinach leaves

½ apple

½ orange, peeled

1 cucumber, cubed

10 raw almonds (soaked overnight)

1 (½ inch) piece fresh ginger root, peeled

2 teaspoons of colostrum

2 tablespoons of chia seeds

2 tablespoons of coconut oil

Place all ingredients in a blender and blend until smooth.

This should make about two 12 oz. (350ml) servings.

Enjoy!

## Healthy Salad Smoothie

1 cup of water

4 ice cubes

½ orange, peeled

1 cup of fresh spinach

½ raw beet, peeled

1/3 cup of baby carrots

1/3 cup of cauliflower floret

1/3 cup of broccoli florets

¼ cup of blueberries

1 stalk of celery

½ lime, peeled

1 tablespoon of honey(optional)

2 tablespoons of coconut oil

2 teaspoons of colostrum

1 tablespoon of chia seeds

10 raw cashew nuts (soaked overnight)

Place all ingredients in a blender and blend until smooth.

This should make about two 12 oz. (350ml) servings.

Enjoy!

## Laura's Banana and Spinach with Oats Smoothie

½ cup of oats

10 raw almonds (soaked overnight)

2 packed handfuls of fresh spinach

1 ripe banana

2 tablespoons of coconut oil

1 tablespoon of maca

1 cup of green tea

6 ice cubes

2 teaspoons of colostrum

1/8 teaspoon of ground cinnamon

Place all ingredients in a blender and blend until smooth.

This should make about two 12 oz. (350ml) servings. Enjoy!

## Green Drink with Aloe Vera Juice smoothie

1 cup of aloe vera juice

½ cup of water

1 cup of green tea

1 handful of baby spinach

1 handful of baby kale

1 cup of baby chard

1 banana

½ cucumber

2 tablespoons of protein powder (optional)

1 teaspoon of ground cinnamon

2 teaspoons of colostrum

2 tablespoons of olive oil

10 raw almonds (soaked overnight)

½ teaspoon of cayenne pepper

Place all ingredients in a blender and blend until smooth. This should make about two 12 oz. (350ml) servings.

Enjoy!

## Veggie, Fruit, and Nut Nutritious Green Smoothie

1 ½ handfuls of baby spinach leaves

1 cup of cubed carrots

½ cup of cubed beet

½ pear, cored and chopped

½ cup of water

1 cup of green tea

½ banana, peeled

¼ cup of walnut halves

10 raw almonds (soaked overnight)

2 tablespoons of coconut oil

1 tablespoon of honey (optional)

½ teaspoon of ground cinnamon

2 teaspoons of chia seeds

2 teaspoons of colostrum

Place all ingredients in a blender and blend until smooth. This should make about two 12 oz. (350ml) servings.

Enjoy!

## Quick Green Smoothie

1 cup of stemmed kale

1 cup of tea

1 banana, peeled

1 handful of barley grass

6 ice cubes

¼ cup of old-fashioned rolled oats

2 tablespoons of coconut oil

10 raw cashew nuts (soaked overnight)

1 tablespoon of flaxseed

1 tablespoon of wheat germ

2 sprigs of fresh parsley, or more to taste

2 teaspoons of colostrum

¼ teaspoon of camu camu

Place all ingredients in a blender and blend until smooth. This should make about two 12 oz. (350ml) servings.

Enjoy!

## Ginger Cabbage Patch Smoothie

1 cup of roughly chopped cabbage
1 cup of red grapes
1 handful of baby kale
1 large carrot, peeled and chopped
1 cup of water
½ cup of ice cubes
2 teaspoons of colostrum
1 tablespoon of fresh ginger
2 tablespoons of coconut oil
Wheat grass, use according to taste
10 raw almonds (soaked overnight)

Place all ingredients in a blender and blend until smooth.

This should make about two 12 oz. (350ml) servings.

Enjoy!

## Liquid Green Platinum smoothie

1 handful of fresh kale
1 packed handful of baby spinach
Fresh parsley (use in small amounts)
1 cup of cubed pineapple
1 ½ cup of chamomile tea
2 tablespoons of coconut oil
2 teaspoons of colostrum
1 teaspoon of chia seeds
10 raw walnuts (soaked overnight)

Place all ingredients in a blender and blend until smooth.

This should make about two 12 oz. (350ml) servings.

Enjoy!

## Wild Pina Colada Green Smoothie

1 ½ cups of fresh diced pineapple
1 cup of coconut water
1 cup of ice cubes

1 cup of chopped dandelion greens

½ cup of shredded unsweetened coconut

10 raw cashew nuts (soaked overnight)

¼ cup of chopped pitted dates, or more to taste

2 tablespoons of coconut oil

2 teaspoons of colostrum

10 raw almonds (soaked overnight)

¼ teaspoon of cayenne pepper

Place all ingredients in a blender and blend until smooth.

This should make about two 12 oz. (350ml) servings.

Enjoy!

## Rosie's Kale Banana Smoothie

1 cup of coconut water or water

1 banana

½ avocado, peeled and pitted

1 ½ handful of packed kale

1 lemon

1 pinch of cayenne pepper

2 tablespoons of coconut oil

2 teaspoons of colostrum

10 raw walnuts (soaked overnight)

Place all ingredients in a blender and blend until smooth.

This should make about two 12 oz. (350ml) servings.

Enjoy!

## Hunter Wellness Mojo smoothie

1 cup of water

½ cup of ice, divided, or as needed

1 (½ inch) piece of fresh ginger

2 teaspoons of ground cinnamon

2 stalks of celery

1 apple

½ cucumber, roughly chopped

4 kale leaves

10 raw walnuts (soaked overnight)

½ handful of fresh spinach, or to taste
¼ cup of mixed salad greens, or to taste
6 fresh mint leaves, or more to taste
2 teaspoons of colostrum
2 tablespoons of olive oil
2 teaspoons of chia seeds

Place all ingredients in a blender and blend until smooth.

This should make about two 12 oz. (350ml) servings.

Enjoy!

## Delicious Cucumber Kale and Blueberry Smoothie

1 large cucumber, diced
1 cup of blueberries
1 cup of vanilla tea
1 cup of ice cubes
1 tablespoon of flaxseeds
2 teaspoons of colostrum
1 teaspoon of cayenne pepper
1 teaspoon of ground ginger
10 raw walnuts (soaked overnight)
2 tablespoons of olive oil

Place all ingredients in a blender and blend until smooth.

This should make about two 12 oz. (350ml) servings.

Enjoy!

## Katie's Beet-Red Raspberry Smoothie

1 cup of fresh raspberries
1 cup of green tea
½ cup of chopped carrot
½ cup of chopped fresh beet
1 lemon, peeled
4 teaspoons of agave nectar(optional)
1 cup of ice cubes
10 raw almonds (soaked overnight)
2 tablespoons of coconut oil
2 teaspoons of colostrum

½ a teaspoon of cayenne pepper

Place all ingredients in a blender and blend until smooth.

This should make about two 12 oz. (350ml) servings.

Enjoy!

## Healthy Daily Smoothie

½ handful of fresh spinach
1 handful of barley grass
¼ cup of fresh blueberries
1 tablespoon of grape seed oil
1 tablespoon of chia seeds
1 tablespoon of flaxseed
10 raw almonds (soaked overnight)
2 teaspoon of colostrum
¼ teaspoon of camu camu
2 tablespoons of coconut oil

Place all ingredients in a blender and blend until smooth.

This should make about two 12 oz. (350ml) servings.

Enjoy!

## Mouthwatering Tomato Basil Smoothie

1 packed handful of fresh spinach leaves
½ large tomato, cut into chunks
½ cup of mango chunks
½ cup of ice cubes
1 cup of green tea
2 teaspoons of coconut oil
2 large fresh basil leaves
10 raw walnuts (soaked overnight)
2 teaspoons of colostrum
2 teaspoons of chia seeds

Place all ingredients in a blender and blend until smooth.

This should make about two 12 oz. (350ml) servings.

Enjoy!

## Japanese Style Pumpkin Banana Tofu Smoothie

1 banana, peeled
1 cup of iced tea
½ cup of water (chilled)
1 cup of pumpkin chunks
½ cup of tofu
10 almonds, or more to taste(soaked overnight)
1 tablespoon of ground cinnamon
2 teaspoons of colostrum
12 teaspoons of cayenne pepper
1 teaspoon of ground nutmeg
2 tablespoons of coconut oil

Place all ingredients in a blender and blend until smooth.

This should make about two 12 oz. (350ml) servings.

Enjoy!

## 'Kalenutsco' Smoothie

1 ½ cups of coconut water
1 ½ packed handful of kale leaves
10 raw walnuts (soaked overnight)
½ cup of shredded sweetened coconut
2 teaspoons of colostrum
2 tablespoons of coconut oil
¼ teaspoon of camu camu

Place all ingredients in a blender and blend until smooth.

This should make about two 12 oz. (350ml) servings.

Enjoy!

## Joanna's Pumpkin Banana Smoothie

1 ½ cups of chamomile tea (chilled)
1 banana, peeled
1 cup of pumpkin chunks
3 dates, pitted
3 ice cubes (optional)
2 tablespoons of chia seeds
2 tablespoons of large flake oats
1 tablespoon of hemp seeds

1 ½ teaspoons of pumpkin pie spice

1 teaspoon of molasses

1 teaspoon of honey (optional)

2 tablespoons of coconut oil

¼ teaspoon of pure vanilla extract

2 teaspoons of colostrum

Wheat grass (use to your taste)

10 raw almonds (soaked overnight)

Place all ingredients in a blender and blend until smooth.

This should make about two 12 Oz. (350ml) servings.

Enjoy!

## Joanna's Carrot with Kale Smoothie

1 large carrot, peeled and diced

½ banana, peeled

2 packed handfuls of kale

½ cup of iced tea

1 cup of cool water

1 tablespoon of ground cinnamon

2 teaspoons of colostrum

1 teaspoon of ground allspice

¼ teaspoon of cayenne pepper

10 raw walnuts (soaked overnight)

2 tablespoons of olive oil

Place all ingredients in a blender and blend until smooth.

This should make about two 12 oz. (350ml) servings.

Enjoy!

---

## Creamy Green smoothie

1 ½ cups of cold water
1 packed handful of baby spinach
½ cup of fresh parsley
½ avocado, peeled and pitted
1 lemon, peeled
2 teaspoons of safflower oil
2 teaspoons of colostrum
½ teaspoon of cayenne pepper
10 raw cashew nuts (soaked overnight)

Place all ingredients in a blender and blend until smooth.

This should make about two 12 Oz. (350ml) servings.

Enjoy!

---

## Blueberry Cucumber Smoothie

1 banana, peeled
1 ½ cucumbers
¾ cup of green tea
8 ice cubes
¼ cup of coconut water
2 tablespoons of blueberry preserves
2 tablespoons of olive oil
2 teaspoons of colostrum
¼ teaspoon of camu camu
10 raw walnuts (soaked overnight)

Place all ingredients in a blender and blend until smooth.

This should make about two 12 Oz. (350ml) servings.

Enjoy!

## Zucchini and Carrot Smoothie

1 zucchini, chopped
1 carrot – peeled and chopped
1 cup of chilled tea
½ cup of coconut water or water
2 tablespoons of rolled oats
2 tablespoons of honey(optional)
1 tablespoon of flaxseeds 2 teaspoons of colostrum
1 teaspoon of Maca
2 teaspoons of coconut oil
10 raw almonds (soaked overnight)

Place all ingredients in a blender and blend until smooth.

This should make about two 12 Oz. (350ml) servings.

Enjoy!

## Green Detox Smoothie

1 cup of green tea
6 ice cubes
2 packed handfuls of fresh spinach leaves
¼ pear, chopped
¼ green apple
¼ avocado
3 broccoli florets
2 teaspoons of colostrum
2 tablespoons of coconut oil
½ teaspoon of cayenne pepper
10 raw almonds (soaked overnight)

Place all ingredients in a blender and blend until smooth.

This should make about two 12 Oz. (350ml) servings.

Enjoy!

## Creamy Pumpkin Pie Smoothie

1  banana, peeled

¾ cup of
green tea
¾ cup of coconut water or water
½ cup of ice, or as desired
¼ cup of pumpkin cubes
½ teaspoon of pumpkin pie spice
2 teaspoons of colostrum
¼ teaspoon of camu camu
2 tablespoons of coconut oil
10 raw cashew nuts (soaked overnight)

Place all ingredients in a blender and blend until smooth.

This should make about two 12 Oz. (350ml) servings.

Enjoy!

## Healthy Pumpkin Smoothie

1 ½ cups of green tea
1 apple
½ frozen banana
1 cup of pumpkin, cubed
3 dates, pitted
3 ice cubes
2 tablespoons of chia seeds
2 tablespoons of large flake oats
1 tablespoon of hemp seeds
1 ½ teaspoons of pumpkin pie spice
1 teaspoon of colostrum
1 teaspoon of honey (optional)
¼ teaspoon of pure vanilla extract
2 tablespoons of coconut oil

Place all ingredients in a blender and blend until smooth.

This should make about two 12 Oz. (350ml) servings.

Enjoy!

## Lisa's Strawberry Lettuce Smoothie

3          cup

s of chopped romaine lettuce

1/3 cup of iced tea, or more as needed

1 cup of coconut water or water

4 ice cubes

4 frozen strawberries, or more to taste

½ banana, cut into chunks

10 raw walnuts (soaked overnight)

¼ teaspoon of vanilla extract, or to taste (optional)

2 teaspoons of colostrum

¼ teaspoon of camu-camu

2 tablespoons of coconut oil

Place all ingredients in a blender and blend until smooth.

This should make about two 12 Oz. (350ml) servings.

Enjoy!

## Jean's Avocado and Carrot with Apple Smoothie

1 ½ (350 ml) cups of cold water

1 apple

2 carrots, cut into chunks

1 lemon, peeled

1 packed handful of kale

10 raw almonds (soaked overnight)

1 (1 inch) piece of fresh ginger root, or more to taste

4 ice cubes

1 avocado, peeled, and pitted

½ teaspoon of cayenne pepper

2 tablespoons of coconut oil

2 teaspoons of colostrum

Place all ingredients in a blender and blend until smooth.

This should make about two 12 oz. (350ml) servings.

Enjoy!

## Cinnamon Apple Healthy Smoothie

1 handful of
baby kale
1 pear, cored and sliced
1 apple, sliced
1 handful of fresh spinach
1 teaspoon ground cinnamon
½ cup of ice
1 cup of green tea
2 tablespoons of coconut oil
2 teaspoons of colostrum
2 teaspoons of chia seeds
10 raw walnuts (soaked overnight)

Place all ingredients in a blender and blend until smooth.

This should make about two 12 Oz. (350ml) servings.

Enjoy!

## Lessee's Lemon Celery Smoothie

1 celery stalk, chopped
½ cucumber, sliced (frozen)
½ apple, chopped
1 cup of iced tea
6 ice cubes
1 packet of stevia (optional)
½ lemon
2 teaspoons of colostrum
1 tablespoon of chia seeds
10 raw almonds (soaked overnight)
2 tablespoons of sunflower oil

Place all ingredients in a blender and blend until smooth.

This should make about two 12 Oz. (350ml) servings.

Enjoy!

## Sweet Green Smoothie

1 ½ cup of
chamomile tea
1 organic banana, preferably frozen
1 bunch of organic broccoli florets (stalk removed)
1 teaspoon of ground cinnamon
¼ teaspoon of camu camu
2 teaspoons of colostrum
1 tablespoon of raw honey or maple syrup(optional)
10 raw almonds (soaked overnight)
2 tablespoons of coconut oil

Place all ingredients in a blender and blend until smooth.
This should make about two 12 Oz. (350ml) servings.
Enjoy!

## Chocolate Mint Green Smoothie

2 packed handful of organic spinach
1 cup of unsweetened coconut water (or water )
1 cup of ice of cubes
½ avocado, pit and skin removed
1 scoop of chocolate protein powder of choice
Several mint leaves
10 raw walnuts (soaked overnight)
1 tablespoon of dark chocolate chips or cacao nibs
Stevia (optional)
2 tablespoons of coconut oil
2 teaspoons of colostrum
½ teaspoons of cayenne pepper
Place all ingredients in a blender and blend until smooth.
This should make about two 12 Oz. (350ml) servings.
Enjoy!

## Green Soothing Smoothie

2 packed
handfuls of fresh spinach
1 cup of cubed cucumber
1 ½ cups of green tea
1 orange, peeled
4 ice cubes
10 raw walnuts (soaked overnight)
2 teaspoons of colostrum
2 tablespoons of coconut oil
¼ teaspoon of cayenne pepper
2 teaspoons of flaxseeds
4 fresh mint leaves, or more to taste

Place all ingredients in a blender and blend until smooth.

This should make about two 12 oz. (350ml) servings.

Enjoy!

## Super Green Super Vibrant Cucumber Apple and Ginger Smoothie

1 small cucumber, cubed
1 packed handful of spinach
1 apple
1 tablespoon of minced ginger
1 lime, peeled
1 tablespoon of honey/agave/maple syrup(optional)
10 raw walnuts (soaked overnight)
2 teaspoons of colostrum
1 cup of water
½ cup of green tea
2 tablespoons of coconut oil
¼ teaspoon of camu camu

Place all ingredients in a blender and blend until smooth.

This should make about two 12 Oz. (350ml) servings.

Enjoy!

## Green Fruity Smoothie

½ orange, peeled

2 generous handfuls of spinach

½ mango peeled and pitted

¼ kiwi, peeled

¼ banana

1 cup of your favorite green tea

1 cup of ice

2 teaspoons of colostrum

2 tablespoons of coconut oil

10 raw almonds (soaked overnight)

2 teaspoons of chia seeds

Place all ingredients in a blender and blend until smooth.

This should make about two 12 Oz. (350ml) servings.

Enjoy!

## Sweet Punch Romaine Lettuce Smoothie

1 cup of water (If you are drinking this straight away, replace this with one cup of ice and add it at the end of blending)

1 cup of chamomile tea

1 banana or 1 cup of mango or 1 small mango

1 apple

1 cup of chopped romaine lettuce, tightly packed

2 tablespoons of pumpkin seeds

½ cup of dried apricots

2 teaspoons of chia seeds

1 cup of oats

10 raw walnuts (soaked overnight)

2 teaspoons of coconut oil

2 teaspoons of colostrum

Place all ingredients in a blender and blend until smooth.

This should make about two 12 Oz. (350ml) servings.

Enjoy!

## Blueberry Avocado Green Smoothie

1 cup of water

1 cup of fresh blueberries

1 small cucumber

½ ripe avocado, pitted and sliced

2 heaping cups of spinach

2 teaspoons of colostrum

10 raw cashew nuts (soaked overnight)

2 tablespoons of coconut oil

2 teaspoons of Maca

1 tablespoon of agave

1 cup of ice

Place all ingredients in a blender and blend until smooth.

This should make about two 12 Oz. (350ml) servings.

Enjoy!

## Aunt Marie's Kale-Ginger Detox Smoothie

½ ripe banana, peeled

½ cup of frozen blueberries

2 teaspoons of ginger, peeled

2 cups of kale leaves, closely packed

1 cup of chamomile tea

6 ice cubes

2 tablespoons of coconut oil

1 tablespoon of chia seeds

1/8 teaspoon of ground cinnamon

2 teaspoons of colostrum

2 teaspoons to 1 tablespoon of raw honey(optional)

10 raw almonds (soaked overnight)

Place all ingredients in a blender and blend until smooth.

This should make about two 12 Oz. (350ml) servings.

Enjoy!

## Healthy Monster Parsley, Kale, and Berry Smoothie

½ cup (packed) of flat-leaf parsley (leaves and stems)
2 packed handfuls of kale leaves (center ribs removed)
½ cup of frozen organic berries (such as strawberries or raspberries)
½ banana
1 teaspoon of ground flaxseed
2 teaspoons of colostrum
2 tablespoons of coconut oil
¼ teaspoon of camu camu
10 raw almonds (soaked overnight)
1 cup of green tea
½ cup of water

Place all ingredients in a blender and blend until smooth.

This should make about two 12 Oz. (350ml) servings.

Enjoy!

## Tropical Cabbage Smoothie

1 cup of coconut water
4 ice cubes
1 lemon
½ large cabbage cubed
½ orange, peeled
2 teaspoons of chia seeds
2 teaspoons of colostrum
2 tablespoons of coconut oil
1 pinch of cayenne pepper
10 raw almonds (soaked overnight)
4 blueberries, or more to taste

Place all ingredients in a blender and blend until smooth.

This should make about two 12 oz. (350ml) servings.

Enjoy!

## Fruity Green Kale-Apple Smoothie

¾ cup of chopped kale, ribs and thick stems removed

1 small stalk of celery, chopped

½ banana

½ apple

½ cup of ice

1 cup of coconut water of green tea

2 teaspoons of colostrum

2 teaspoons of chia seeds

½ teaspoon of cayenne pepper

2 teaspoons of coconut oil

1 fresh lemon, peeled

10 raw almonds(soaked overnight)

Place all ingredients in a blender and blend until smooth.

This should make about two 12 oz. (350ml) servings.

Enjoy!

# IMPORTANT MEDICAL WARNING & DISCLAIMER

Breast-feeding or pregnant women should abstain from any type of detox program. These toxins can be transferred to the infant.

The information in this book is not intended as medical advice, or to replace a one-on-one relationship with a qualified health-care professional. It is intended as a sharing of knowledge and information from personal research and experience.

Please make your own health care decisions based upon your research and in partnership with a qualified health care professional.

Always work directly with a qualified medical professional before attempting to treat any illness or medical condition with diet and lifestyle, or when changing or discontinuing any prescription medications. Always ask your doctor before making any changes in diet when you have an existing medical condition. Always check with your doctor before starting any new diet or fitness program.

The nutritional information provided in this book is approximated and based on a 2000-calorie diet. Nutritional data was obtained from the USDA National Nutrient Database for Standard Reference, Release 22. Actual nutritional values may vary based on factors including, but not limited to, size of produce, freshness, processing, geographic region, and season.

# ABOUT THE AUTHORS

## Marcus D. Norman
### Biography

Marcus D. Norman is an entrepreneur, world adventurer, health fanatic and family man. He was not always that way, and in his young 20s, he was a verified couch potato and tells us that he loved junk food and movies, and that a regular diet of large Snickers bars and can Coca-Cola was his staple diet for the day!

Marcus D. Norman had found himself with two supposedly incurable diseases. He was told by numerous doctors that he would have to take medication and live with these conditions for the rest of his life. That was the fuel that lit his fire to learn all he could about how to have optimal health and eliminate diseases from his life.

He is very passionate about sharing his knowledge and his experience on how he turned it around and how you can do the same.

He gets very thrilled when he sets another person free from drugs and disease.

He discovered yoga over 30 years ago, and also discovered the enormous benefits of diet. He spends most of his time in the United States of America and Thailand. He has studied with some of the world's best instructors for health and well-being, Anthony Carlisi, David Swenson, Tias Little and Pete Egoscue to name a few.

Some of the activities he enjoys are; scuba, sailing, snow skiing, and hiking mountains. He has climbed the peaks of Machu Picchu in Cusco Peru (14,050 ft. above sea level) and has also done a 3-day hike on five different occasions. He states that it is like winning a Gold Medal, and an incredible experience to reach this ancient city. He has also traveled three different times on a 5,000mile motorcycle trip through Mexico, Flying Hang glider, Ultralights, Paragliders, Sailplanes, and Cycling.

He has lived and traveled to 18 countries, appreciates other cultures and customs, and he really loves to be outdoors. His diet is mostly veggie juices, brown rice, fruits, vegetables, seafood and he is crazy for Thai food!!!

*Basic Life Philosophy...*

*"LIFE IS GOOD!"*

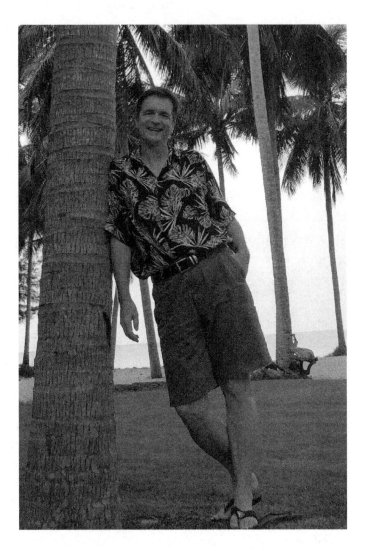

TEN-DAY GREEN SUPERFOOD SMOOTHIE CLEANSE

# Dr. George Della Pietra N.D.

# My Biography

There are two typical reasons why somebody would approach a career in the medical field 1) to make as much money as possible, or 2) their own experience with diseases as a patient, often for a long period, and therefore, actually the desire to heal oneself. My career was obviously not a typical one, as I was never interested in money at all, and my health was excellent for as long as I can think. Even more, I had two older brothers being medical doctors already and therefore, a very clear understanding of what western medicine is able to achieve and what not. This was of absolutely no interest to me. I chose to be a musician and journalist instead first.

However, at the age of 30, I had a look back at an extremely happy, and as I feel, very privileged life. The absence of ever having to see a doctor made me simply want to "give something back." Since I am not religious, there was no God I could be thankful to, so I decided to give back to humanity and began to study all kinds of medicine I thought would be useful to help other people to get cured of any kind of severe diseases. This includes Western Medicine (only for "communication reasons"), Chinese Medicine, Naturopathy including all kinds of manual therapies and a focus on Energetic Medicine ("spiritual" as well as using modern western equipment). I collected a couple of diplomas and certificates, but, to be honest, was actually never really interested in them – I always studied to broaden my horizon, and not to get a piece of paper in the end.

Being lucky as usual, I opened my first naturopathic clinic in Switzerland, and was extremely busy helping to improve the health and life quality of my patients, and among them was many cases of cancer, AIDS and other lifethreatening diseases or syndromes. Unfortunately, I found out that most cures which really work are either illegal or at least borderline. So, I decided it was better I didn't work as a practitioner anymore. Consequently, I moved to Thailand for a decade, set up and ran some of the best spas in Asia – believing a beautiful and healthy environment does really support cures and prevention of all kinds. Back in Europe, I focus on projects like this book, my new company www.zuerihomemassage.com and as soon as time permits, the setup of the independent health platform www.thenaturallibrary.com - coming soon.

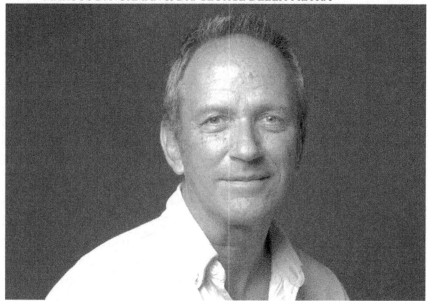

Dr. George Della Pietra N.D.
Zürich Switzerland